GERIATRICS, GERONTOLOGY AND ELDERLY ISSUES

IS AGING A DISEASE?

UNTANGLING THE RELATIONSHIP

Geriatrics, Gerontology and Elderly Issues

Additional books and e-books in this series can be found on Nova's website under the Series tab.

GERIATRICS, GERONTOLOGY AND ELDERLY ISSUES

IS AGING A DISEASE?

UNTANGLING THE RELATIONSHIP

MICHAEL A. SINGER

nova
Medicine & Health
New York

NOTICE TO THE READER

Library of Congress Cataloging-in-Publication Data

ISBN: 978-1-53615-509-9
Library of Congress Control Number: 2019940470

Published by Nova Science Publishers, Inc. † New York

CONTENTS

PREFACE

Each species has its own characteristic aging trajectory coded by a species-specific developmental program. This developmental program is triggered at the time of fertilization, hence aging begins at conception. Within a species, there is considerable between individual variations in the aging phenotype due to the plasticity of the developmental process and its inherent stochasticity. The evolution of a species is due to genetic changes in its underlying developmental program and when enough genetic changes have accumulated a new species emerges with its own characteristic aging phenotype. Therefore, speciation and aging are linked processes. Over the evolutionary course of the human lineage, culture has been an important driver of evolutionary change. Culture is not restricted to the human lineage but only humans have evolved cumulative culture; the transmission of modified cultural practices across generations. Early cultural innovations such as toolmaking, agriculture and dairy farming had a utilitarian function. However, over the past 100-150 years there has been a significant change in the pace and nature of cultural innovations. Although many cultural innovations still have a utilitarian function, a new category of cultural innovations has emerged that have "entertainment" functions in the domains of social communication and information transfer. In addition, cultural practices by the tobacco, food and technological industries have been used to modify population behaviors, physiology and beliefs. Over the past 50 – 75 years there has emerged so called chronic non-infectious diseases which occurrence parallels the development of these new cultural innovations and practices. In addition, culture has now become the primary driver of human evolution. In answer to the question posed by the title of this book, aging is not a disease and diseases are cultural constructs used to define variants in the aging process.

INTRODUCTION

Why write another book about aging, given how many have already been penned? There is a specific purpose, however, for writing this book. Over the past one hundred years, particularly in developed countries, there has been a doubling of average human life expectancy. However, health span, disease-free lifespan, has not increased to the same extent as life extension (Partridge et al., 2018). The result is that developed countries must now deal with a growing population of aging individuals suffering from late-life diseases. How is this looming problem to be managed? Strategies to address this issue must be developed within a framework that defines the nature of the aging process, what constitutes a disease and the relationship between aging and diseases.

Currently, the favored view is that aging is a time dependent accumulation of somatic damage resulting from the diminished strength of natural selection that occurs after attainment of reproductive maturity. Within this framework, organisms preferentially invest resources into somatic maintenance and repair in early life but let these mechanisms lapse after reproductive maturity is reached. A number of dysregulated molecular processes have been identified as being responsible for this late life accumulated somatic damage and these dysregulated molecular processes have been termed the "Hallmarks of Aging" (Lopez-Otin et al., 2013).

Disease is a well-used term but difficult to define. At the present time, a disease is considered to be a pathologic process expressed as a collection of symptoms and physical manifestations specific to that designated disease. A disease has the property of being alien to the individual in that a pathologic process has usurped normal physiological processes.

These current concepts of aging and disease will bias how we regard the connection between aging and diseases. Many consider aging to be the major risk factor for chronic non-infectious diseases (Partridge et al., 2018) while others have extended this view and consider the aging process itself to be a disease (Bulterijs et al., 2015). These particular concepts of aging and disease will set specific research agendas and in addition, will raise certain expectations within the public. Words with their associated meanings can be powerful instruments. If we label aging as the prime risk factor for non-infectious diseases, will the public believe that if the dysregulated processes underlying aging can be corrected then diseases will be cured and that aging will be abolished? In light of the highly technological nature of modern human culture, and the significant increases in human lifespan that has resulted from advanced medical interventions, are these public expectations unrealistic?

In this book I am going to present an alternative view; aging is not a disease nor should it be regarded as primarily a major risk factor for chronic non-infectious diseases and diseases should be considered as simply variations of the aging process.

In the paradigm to be discussed in this book, each species has an evolved specific aging pattern because aging as a process is embedded or coded in the developmental program of that species. Within a species there are considerable between-individual variations in the aging process with the boundaries of that variation constrained by the developmental program itself. For humans, there are two forms of non-genetic inheritance that have become the primary drivers of evolutionary change; cultural and ecological inheritance (niche construction). However these two forms of non-genetic inheritance do not act in a unidirectional mode. Culture and niche construction are not only "products" of evolution but also "causes" of evolution and hence they represent examples of reciprocal causation. Human populations pass culture and modified environmental spaces to succeeding generations but at the same time cultural practices and modified environmental spaces change the natural selective forces acting on these populations; in essence forming a feedback loop. For example, the very technological devices and practices that we have created to solve specific problems have the potential through the action of reciprocal causation to modify the (natural) selective forces acting on us and thus change our own evolutionary trajectory. It is no coincidence that the explosion of chronic non-infectious diseases over the past 100 to 150 years parallels the rapid evolution of human culture and niche construction.

I will also explore the disease concept, its historical roots and its relationship to cultural beliefs and scientific thought. The disease concept is a cultural construct. Since aging varies extensively across individuals, a disease simply becomes a manifestation of the extreme variations in biology that exists between individuals. We have great difficulty defining what is normal for human physiological traits. We generally use statistical tools to define a trait's normal range as being within two standard deviations on either side of a mean value. This definition of what constitutes a normal range is clearly arbitrary and thereby creates an arbitrary range for what is abnormal i.e., a disease.

If the aging process is part of a species developmental program and if a disease represents an extreme variation of a species aging process, then diseases cannot be cured and aging cannot be abolished. The management of aging and so-called diseases must be framed in terms of more realistic goals than is currently the practice.

In this introduction I have briefly introduced a few of the implications associated with different concepts of aging and disease. In the following sections, I will discuss in more depth the consequences of aging envisioned to be a process embedded in a species-specific developmental program and non-infectious diseases as being extreme variations in between-individual biology. From a human and global perspective, the powerful influence of culture and niche construction cannot be overemphasized and this topic will be explored in some depth. How we humans manage aging and manage so called non-infectious diseases will ultimately depend on our understanding of these processes.

Chapter 1

AGING

BACKGROUND

It is essential, at the start, to define the meaning of concepts and terms used in this book (Kampourakis and Stern, 2018; Moore, 2013). I will use the terms aging and senescence interchangeably. Within the classical evolutionary framework, aging is defined as an age-specific increase in mortality and/or an age-specific decrease in reproductive capacity (Singer, 2018 b). This definition has been expanded to include several subcategories. Negligible senescence is defined as no measurable decline in reproductive success with age and/or no measurable increase in mortality with age. Even the notion of negative senescence has been proposed and is defined as an age-specific decrease in mortality accompanied by an age-specific increase in reproductive success. These classical evolutionary definitions of aging are based upon the idea that natural selection weakens after attainment of reproductive maturity thereby allowing biological damage to accumulate. The implication is that aging is a lifecycle stage that occurs after reproductive maturity is achieved and that aging can be defined by measures of age-specific mortality and age-specific fecundity.

I favor a more general definition of aging as a species-specific time dependent decline in the physiological functions of an organism ultimately resulting in death of that organism. This definition underscores that the aging pattern differs between species and does not restrict aging to a particular period of the lifecycle or restrict the aging process to measures of fertility and mortality rate. For example, the aging pattern of worker honey bees, which lack reproductive capability, is set by their social function (Munch and Amdam, 2010). The classical evolutionary definition does not fit this pattern. Also this general definition does not stipulate a rate for the aging process i.e., as to whether it is gradual or rapid. As will become apparent, aging actually begins at the time of fertilization which event triggers a species-specific developmental program.

It is important to study the aging of a species within the context of its natural ecological niche, ecosystem and the multiple interactions between diverse species that characterize its ecosystem (Singer, 2018 b). A case in point is that of Hydra, a small fresh water polyp belonging to the phylum Cnidaria. In controlled laboratory settings this organism appears to be immortal. However, in the wild, hydras subjected to fluctuations in food supply, water temperatures and organism density display signs of aging and have a lifespan of only a few months (Singer, 2016).

Because a species evolves within a specific ecological niche and an ecosystem comprising other diverse interacting species, it is clear that aging cannot be studied as an isolated phenotypic trait (Singer, 2016; Singer, 2018 a). Furthermore, the aging process must be understood within the broader context of the process of speciation.

AGING IN THE WILD; SPECIES SPECIFICITY

Aging in the Wild

In the 1950s the predominant view was that in the wild, animal survival was so short that senescence would not be observed. This prediction was based upon the concept that since the force of natural selection weakened with age, deleterious mutations would accumulate in older individuals and be manifest as senescence in late life. Since most wild animals did not achieve a long lifespan because of predation and other extrinsic factors, senescence would not be observed. However, a number of studies have been published documenting senescence in the wild.

Nussey et al., (2013) collected empirical evidence for senescence in wild animals. Senescence was generally measured as a decline in age-related survival probability and/or age-related decline in reproductive performance, although in some of the collected studies age-related declines in other traits were also measured. These investigators found 340 studies involving 175 species that recorded the occurrence of senescence. The main point of this study was to document that aging (senescence) was most likely universal in wild animals and to dispel the notion that animals in the wild did not live long enough to display aging. Nussey et al., (2013), however, did not comment as to whether different species showed different aging patterns.

Roach and Carey (2014) also looked at the biology of aging in the wild. They found, similar to Nussey et al., (2013), that senescence was quite prevalent in the wild. However, they made the interesting observation that in some species the multiple traits contributing to the aging phenotype, did not all decline at the same time or with the same rate. In addition, plants in particular had a diversity of lifespans and patterns of aging.

Although, these observations of Nussey et al., (2013) and Roach and Carey (2014) confirmed that the aging phenotype was most likely present in all species in the wild, they did not infer whether aging patterns were species-specific. This question was addressed in a study reported by Jones et al., (2014).

Species Specificity

Jones et al., (2014) collected data on the aging patterns of numerous species; 11 mammals, 12 non-mammalian vertebrates, 10 invertebrates, 12 vascular plants and a green alga. Jones et al., (2014) used as their definition of aging, age-specific mortality and age-specific fertility rates i.e., the classical evolutionary definition. For each species, relative mortality and relative fertility were calculated by dividing age-specific rates by the weighted mean for the whole adult population sampled. The age range used for these calculations was the adult lifespan defined as starting at the mean age of reproductive maturation and ending when only 5% of adults were still alive. This method allowed the investigators to compare species with widely different lifespans... Their graphed data showed an incredible variation in the trajectories of mortality and fertility across these 46 diverse species; each species appeared to have evolved its own unique pattern.

Jones et al., (2014) used a methodology which allowed for comparison of aging patterns across the tree of life involving species with a wide range of lifespans. However, studies that have focused on smaller groups of species also underscore the species-specificity of the aging process.

One would expect phylogenetically related species to have similar aging patterns. Bronikowski et al., (2011) described aging patterns in seven non-human primate species. Aging was measured as age-specific mortality using two parameters. An initial adult mortality rate (IMR) was defined as the probability of death at onset of adulthood and rate of aging (RoA) was defined as the rate of increase in age-specific mortality with advancing age. The non-human primate data were compared to published data on humans.

All seven species, plus humans, showed a general pattern of high infant mortality, followed by a juvenile period of low mortality and then an extended period of increasing age-specific mortality during midlife through to later life. Bronikowski et al., (2011) focused specifically on the mid to late life period using the two parameters defined in the preceding paragraph. Values for both parameters, IMR and RoA, were low in humans which accounted for our exceptional longevity. Plots of RoA versus IMR for both females and males of all seven non-human primate species and humans showed four distinct groupings of IMR and three significant groupings for RoA. Hence, the data indicated that these related species show distinguishable aging phenotypes. Furthermore, the investigators noted that the species groupings of IMR and RoA showed no relationship to phylogeny implying that the aging phenotypes across these eight species were not constrained by phylogeny but evolved in response to selection pressures at the species or local population level. In addition, within species comparisons revealed that both IMR and RoA varied substantially among populations within a species.

In a more recent study, the same group of investigators (Alberts et al., 2013) compared reproductive aging and mortality in females of the same seven non-human primate species. Females belonging to the Dobe!Kung population, pre-industrial hunter-foragers living in the Kalahari Desert of southern Africa, were used as a human comparison group. Two parameters were used in the analysis; computed actuarial estimates of age-specific mortality probabilities and age at which each female underwent fertility completion. A female's last birth was considered to represent fertility completion if she survived a prescribed interval following her last live birth without experiencing another live birth. Age-specific probability of fertility completion was used as a measure of reproductive senescence as opposed to cessation of reproduction due to death of the female.

In all seven non-human primate species and the human group, the probability of death increased with advancing age. In four of the non-human primate species the occurrence of fertility completion could not be determined because very few individuals met the criteria. In the other three species, the initial rate of age-specific reproductive senescence (probability of fertility completion) was significantly lower than the initial rate of age-specific mortality but the rate of reproductive senescence increased faster with advancing age than that for mortality. The two lines intersected at the time of death (mortality probability 100%) indicating that it is very difficult to distinguish between cessation of reproduction due to senescence and cessation of reproduction due to death of the female.

In contrast, for the Dobe!Kung the lines defining the rates of age-specific reproductive senescence and age-specific mortality were approximately parallel and both increased with advancing age. The reproductive senescence line was above that for mortality. Reproductive senescence achieved a probability of 100% many years before that of death. In fact, the modal ages of death and reproductive cessation in this human population were 79.25 years and 41.0 years respectively.

In summary, non-human female primates and female humans manifest an increasing probability of reproductive senescence and mortality with advancing age. However, in non-human female primates the actual occurrence of reproductive senescence is exceedingly low and in most cases, cessation of reproduction is due to death and not senescence. In female humans, the occurrence of reproductive senescence is much higher and many individuals experience a prolonged survival period after cessation of reproduction. Alberts et al., (2013) noted that in non-human female primates a small percentage of individuals do experience post reproductive years; on a population level, about 1-6% of adult female years lived were post cessation of reproduction. This measure is termed post reproductive representation and on a population level is defined as the proportion of adult years lived which are post reproductive. In comparison, for the Dobe!Kung population about 42.5% of adult female years lived were post cessation of reproduction. Hence, among primates, female humans are unique in experiencing a lifespan that greatly exceeds the reproductive period. However, humans are not the only mammals displaying this particular aging pattern.

Previous comparative studies have shown that female members of only three species of mammals, humans, killer whales and short-finned pilot whales were known to display a significant post reproductive lifespan (Ellis et al., 2018). Ellis et al., (2018) recently added two more mammalian species to this list. These investigators used anatomical data, age-specific counts of ovarian corpora, to measure the age related life history of reproductive senescence in sixteen species of cetaceans. These data were fitted to age-specific measures of survival to estimate post reproductive lifespan. Post reproductive lifespan was represented as the percentage of adult female years, in the study population, being lived by post reproductive females (post reproductive representation). In non-human female primates, as previously described, this percentage is 1-6% of adult years lived and in the pre-industrial Dobe!Kung female population the value is 42.5%. Ten of the sixteen cetacean species showed a decline in reproductive activity with age but in only three did females display a significant post reproductive lifespan. These three species and their post reproductive representations were; beluga whales 27%, narwhals 24% and short-finned pilot whales 15%. A phylogenetic analysis revealed that in these toothed whales, post reproductive lifespan evolved independently three times; once in the common ancestor of beluga and narwhal, once in the short-finned pilot whale lineage and once in the killer whale lineage.

The evolution of a pronged post reproductive lifespan in females is an unusual aging pattern observed in only a few select mammalian species. The evolution of this particular reproductive aging pattern appears to be driven by changes in local kin relatedness between members of the population across the lifespan (Ellis et al., 2018). In addition, older post reproductive females can increase their inclusive fitness by aiding other members of the group to reproduce through grandmother and mother benefits. Johnstone and Cant (2019) reviewed the selective pressures that appear to be responsible for the evolution of a prolonged post reproductive period in a few mammalian species. Regardless, with respect to the topic of this book, a long post reproductive lifespan is another example of an unusual form of species-specific aging that would be coded in the developmental program of that particular mammalian species.

Another species with an unusual aging pattern is the naked mole rat which is a species in the order Rodentia (Buffenstein, 2005). An allometric regression of maximum species lifespans (MSLP) versus body mass for rodents reveals the naked mole rat to be an outlier with a very long MSLP of close to 30 years. This species also displays negligible senescence. Naked mole rats are fossorial and groups live in extensive mazes of subterranean tunnels. This species is eusocial and colonies show a division of labor including that of reproductive function. A colony, mean size of 75 animals, generally contains a single dominant breeding female and one to three breeding males. Unlike eusocial insects in which the queen lives longer than workers, breeding and non-breeding naked mole rats appear to have similar lifespans.

What factors account for the extreme longevity of naked mole rats? Most studies focus on unusual features of the biology of this species as an explanation. However, the biology of the naked mole rat evolved within the context of its ecological niche and its social interactions not the reverse. This question has been addressed by Williams and Shattuck (2015) and Healy (2015). In both studies, maximum lifespan was compared in 440 ground-dwelling mammals. This group was subdivided into terrestrial (n = 339) or fossorial (n = 101) and eusocial (n = 17) or non-eusocial (n = 423). Comparisons between terrestrial/fossorial and eusocial/non-eusocial were performed with control for body mass and phylogenetic relatedness. The results indicated that both eusociality and a fossorial habitat were significant factors driving the longevity of the naked mole rat. Interestingly Williams and Shattuck (2015) point out that human populations display overlapping generations, reproductive skew and cooperative breeding and although humans are not eusocial in the strict sense these features may help account for the longevity of our species.

Another group of animals with an unusual aging pattern are tardigrades. These are tiny aquatic complex multicellular animals with more than a 1,000 species reported (Hashimoto et al., 2016). Some species, particularly those living in limnoterrestrial habitats can enter a contracted dehydrated state when subjected to extreme water deprivation. These dehydrated tardigrades can withstand extremes in abiotic conditions; extreme temperatures, high pressure, exposure to high doses of irradiation and exposure to space in a low earth orbit (Hashimoto et al., 2016; Sloan et al., 2017). The ecology, lifespan and reproductive senescence of tardigrades have been examined and the genome of one of the more stress-tolerant tardigrade species has been sequenced.

Tardigrades have a symmetrical body plan with four pairs of legs that terminate in claws or sucking discs (Nelson, 2002). They are very small with adult body sizes in the range of 250 micrometres. They have a complete digestive system and a hemocoel type fluid filled body cavity which serves respiratory and circulatory functions. Reproductive modes include sexual reproduction and parthenogenesis. They have a nervous system consisting of a dorsal brain and ventral nerve cord. Tardigrades are classified into two main taxonomic groups based upon morphologic features; character of claws, cuticle, cephalic appendages and reproductive structures.

Although tardigrades live in marine, freshwater and terrestrial habitats, most species are terrestrial (Nelson, 2002). Within the terrestrial environment, tardigrades occupy moist habitats such as soil, leaf litter and mosses. To be active, they must be surrounded by a film of water. When environmental conditions become adverse e.g., freezing, desiccation, low oxygen tension, tardigrades can enter a contracted dehydrated state of reduced or absent metabolism, growth, reproduction and aging. When in such a state, tardigrades are extremely resistant to extremes of temperature, pressure and ionizing radiation. There is little known about optimal conditions for growth and the role of predators, competition and parasitism in determining tardigrade population densities and diversity.

Tsujimoto et al., (2016) studied lifespan and reproductive behavior in the tardigrade species, Acutuncus antarcticus. This species was originally collected from East Antarctica and maintained in the laboratory. This species reproduces through automictic parthenogenesis. Sixty-eight juveniles were studied under standard laboratory conditions. Survival and reproductive behavior were monitored. The latter included; egg production (timing and clutch size), time to egg hatching and hatching success.

Mean and median lifespans were 69.2 and 65 days but there was considerable between individual variations. The minimum to maximum lifespan across the 68 individuals was 12 to 162 days. Reproductive traits also showed extensive between individual variations; minimum to maximum for total number of oviposition events per individual 0-17, total number of eggs per individual 0-97, age at first oviposition 6-11 (days) and days from last oviposition to death 1-54 (days). Individual minimum to maximum for oviposition characteristics were; clutch size 1.4-6.5, oviposition interval 5-11 (days), time to hatching 7.6-9 (days) and hatching success 85.7-100%. In general, clutch size, oviposition interval and hatching success showed very little decline with advancing age. Most individuals continued to reproduce throughout their entire lifespan.

A. antarcticus resides in both terrestrial and freshwater habitats in the Antarctic. This environment is characterized by extremely low temperatures, limited water availability and a short growing season. Minimal reproductive senescence plus the capacity to enter a dehydrated low metabolic state under very adverse environmental conditions appear to be some of the adaptations that have allowed this species to live in this particularly harsh environment.

The life traits and tolerance of R. varieornatus to extreme environmental conditions have been examined under laboratory conditions (Horikawa et al., 2008). This species has a mean life span of 35 days (minimum to maximum 13-87 days), somewhat shorter than that of A. antarcticus. The population studied appeared to have oviposition events throughout the entire lifespan although the number of eggs per individual per day was greater in younger compared to older individuals. Desiccation tolerance was tested in juveniles and adults. Tardigrades were desiccated for 24 hours and preserved in this state for 10 days. Then the dry tardigrades were rehydrated and checked for viability. Juveniles and adults had equal survival (about 95%) following 10 days of desiccation. Horikawa et al., (2008) also assessed survival of these tardigrades after exposure to extreme environments. For each stressor, hydrated tardigrades were compared to desiccated animals. The stressors included heat at 90°C, cold at -196°C, ionizing radiation and exposure to acetonitrile, an organic solvent. Heat and acetonitrile exposure killed all hydrated tardigrades whereas in both cases over 90% of desiccated animals survived. About 20% of hydrated animals survived the cold stressor compared to over 90% of dry animals. Both hydrated and dry animals had equivalent survival to ionizing radiation, over 80%. R. varieornatus is a species that is very tolerant of extreme environmental conditions and relatively easy to maintain in a laboratory setting. These characteristics made this species a good candidate for genome sequencing.

Hashimoto et al., (2016) sequenced the genome of Ramazzottius varieornatus, a very stress resistant species. Previously published data had suggested that the tardigrade genome was almost 20% of foreign origin via extensive horizontal gene transfer but Hashimoto et al., (2016) showed that this finding was probably the result of contamination. In the genome of R. varieornatus there was actually less than 1.2% of foreign gene content and about 41% of genes appeared to be unique to the tardigrade genome. Several stress related gene families, superoxide dismutases and MRE 11

(MRE 11 protein is involved in repair of DNA double stranded breaks), were expanded while several other stress response pathways were missing, including ones responsive to hypoxia and ones that activated the mTOR pathway.

As noted, tardigrade species such as R. varieornatus can enter a low metabolic water contracted state which is highly resistant to extremes of heat and cold for example. Hashimoto et al., (2016) identified a number of tardigrade unique proteins including members of the CAHS (cytosolic-abundant heat soluble proteins) and SAHS (secretory-abundant heat soluble proteins) families. SAHS and CAHS proteins change their conformation when subjected to water deficient conditions and have been proposed to protect biomolecules during desiccation. The investigators identified 16 CAHS and 13 SAHS genes in the assembly.

R. varieornatus is extremely tolerant to high dose radiation and Hashimoto et al., (2016) detected a unique DNA-associated protein, termed damage suppressor protein (Dsup) that is involved in the resistance of this species to radiation. The protective action of Dsup is thought to be through the formation of as complex between Dsup and DNA. To test the actions of Dsup, Hashimoto et al., (2016) generated a human cell line expressing Dsup. When this cell line was exposed to ionizing radiation, there were fewer single-stranded and double-stranded DNA breaks compared to the same cell line not expressing Dsup. In addition, the cell line expressing Dsup had a higher survival rate (measured as changes in morphology and proliferative capacity) following ionizing radiation compared to the same cell line not expressing Dsup.

The genome of R. varieornatus contains unique genes that encode proteins conferring the capacity of this tardigrade to resist extreme environmental conditions. Some of these proteins protect biomolecules from the effects of desiccation and a unique DNA-complexing protein shields DNA from the damaging effects of ionizing radiation. In addition, at least in the laboratory, tardigrades show negligible reproductive senescence; this organism appears to be capable of reproduction throughout its lifespan. How do we account for these life traits; negligible aging, capacity to enter states highly resistant to extreme abiotic stressors and tolerance to ionizing radiation? I would propose that a highly specific developmental program is the basis of these unusual features of tardigrades.

The comprehensive study of aging across the tree of life by Jones et al., (2014) and the aging phenotypes I have described for more limited groups of species highlight the sheer diversity of aging patterns that are observed across species. What mechanism could account for such an observation? I propose that this observation is most easily accounted for by a process that is species-specific and the most reasonable candidate for such a process is the developmental program that is specific to each species and in essence makes that species what it is. The concept that aging is embedded in species-specific developmental programs connects aging to the process of speciation. New species emerge from existing species when a new developmental program has evolved. This evolutionary process does not occur in isolation but within the context of ecological niches and ecosystems. An ecosystem is not a random collection of species but a regulated hierarchical biological organization comprised of interacting communities of diverse species. (For example, Hatton et al., (2015) observed a scaling relationship between predator biomass and prey biomass that applied to more than 2,260 ecosystems, both aquatic and terrestrial). The evolution of existing species and the emergence of new species occur under the guidance of multilevel selection.

Within the scientific community, conceptualizing the evolution of an aging phenotype has been approached from a different perspective than conceptualizing the evolution of other phenotypes. Comments advanced about aging in a recent paper help illustrate this point. Dong et al., (2016) used epidemiological data to estimate maximum human lifespan and on the basis of their analysis, these investigators concluded that human longevity had a fixed ceiling with a natural limit of about 115 years. In the discussion about a mechanism to account for such a maximum lifespan in humans, Dong et al., (2016) stated that; "The idea that ageing is a purposeful, programmed series of events that evolved under the direct force of natural selection to cause death has now been all but discredited." Yet, they postulated that the natural limit to human longevity was an inadvertent byproduct of early life fixed genetic programs such as development, growth and reproduction. However, is not the proposal that a maximum lifespan for humans is a by-product of early life genetic programs, the same as ascribing human maximum lifespan to being coded within a human species-specific developmental program?

The developmental program of a species codes for the specific morphology, biology and behaviors that are unique to that species. When a sperm and an egg of a giraffe unite to form a zygote, a developmental program is triggered that gives rise to a fully formed giraffe with its characteristic shape, biology and behaviors. Similarly, when a human sperm and egg unite, the developmental program of the zygote gives rise to a recognizable human. Of course there is extensive within species variations; not all individual giraffes are the same and not all individual humans are the same. However, a species developmental program is specific enough that a giraffe's program does not form a human and the human developmental program does not form a giraffe. The aging phenotype is one of the traits coded by a species developmental program and so is a species sleep behaviors. As a digression, I will describe the diversity of sleep behaviors across species as an analogy to the diversity of aging patterns across species. The point is that aging as a species-specific phenotype has evolved as part of developmental programs in the same way as have other phenotypes such as species-specific sleep patterns.

My choice of sleep as an analogous phenotype is not entirely arbitrary. Both aging and sleep are widespread in occurrence and evolutionarily ancient. But, these two phenotypes are also connected. Age-related changes have been described in the sleep state of humans, in such features as timing, duration and architecture (e.g., proportion of REM sleep) (Espiritu, 2008). However, disentangling how the specific effects of aging compared to the effects of our modern day culture have changed ancestral pre-industrial human sleep patterns is still problematical.

Sleep Patterns across Species; A Phenotype Analogous to Aging

Just as it was important to define the term aging, it is equally important to define what constitutes a sleep state. A sleep state is defined by a combination of behavioral criteria (Lesku and Ly, 2017; Joiner, 2016). These behaviors include; decreased responsiveness to stimulation, rapid reversibility to an awake condition and homeostatic regulation. The latter refers to the observation that an animal kept awake will, when sleep is allowed to proceed, sleep longer and more deeply, thus making up for lost sleep. Since sleep constitutes a state of reduced responsiveness, this state can limit a number of other behaviors such as defense against predation, foraging for food and mating. However, sleep can be plastic within the context of different ecological settings. Examples of this plasticity include; suppression of sleep activity in male polygynous pectoral sandpipers during mating and suppression of sleep activity in white-crowned sparrows during migration (Joiner, 2016).

In addition, unihemispheric sleep has been described in mammals, birds and possibly reptiles (Manoach and Stickgold, 2016). Unihemispheric sleep in aquatic mammals allows these animals to continue swimming and to surface for air while asleep. In birds during long migratory flights, unihemispheric sleep allows them to migrate and maintain vigilance. Ducks in the outer perimeter of a group settled near a pond, maintain watchfulness through unihemispheric sleep while those in the center of the group have "normal" bihemispheric sleep.

In humans there is evidence that asymmetric hemispheric sleep rather than true unihemispheric sleep can occur (Tamaki et al., 2016). Humans often experience disrupted sleep in a new environment. This phenomenon has been observed, for example, on the first night of a laboratory sleep study, so called first night effect. Tamaki et al., (2016) compared measurements made during the first and second nights of a laboratory sleep study. The data revealed asymmetry in slow wave activity between the two hemispheres but only on night one. In their experiments, the left hemisphere was not sleeping as deeply as the right hemisphere. How could they explain these results? They tested the hypothesis that reduced sleep intensity in the left hemisphere was due to maintained vigilance in this hemisphere on night one of a new environment. Experimental testing supported this hypothesis; the more awake left hemisphere acted as a night watch in an unfamiliar environment to protect the sleeper.

Sleep patterns have been found to be quite diverse across the tree of life. Two types of sleep have been described; rapid-eye-movement sleep (REM) and non REM sleep (Peever and Fuller, 2017). Initially, REM sleep was distinguished on the basis of rapid eye movements produced by contractions of oculomotor muscles, but it is now known that REM sleep has other defining physiological, behavioral and brain electrical activity features. REM sleep has been identified in terrestrial mammals, birds, reptiles and some aquatic invertebrates (Peever and Fuller, 2017). Across species there is considerable variation in frequency and duration of REM sleep. Horses, giraffes and elephants spend less than one hour each day in REM sleep while ferrets, platypuses and house cats spend three to eight hours each day in REM sleep. In mice, REM sleep periods occur every 10 to 15 minutes while in humans the frequency is every 90 to 120 minutes. Among primates humans have the shortest duration of sleep (REM plus non REM phases) but the highest proportion of REM sleep (Nunn et al., 2016).

A sleep state has been described in insects as well (Helfrich-Forster, 2018). In honey bees sleep deprivation at night impairs the precision of waggle-dance signaling and reduces the probability of successful return to the hive the following day.

Sleep has been documented in the cnidarian jellyfish Cassiopea (Nath et al., 2017). The neurons in this organism are formed into a diffuse radially symmetric net. Hence, the observations of Nath et al., (2017) indicate that the sleep state arose prior to the evolution of an organized central nervous system.

Although sleep subserves many neurobiological functions (Lesku and Ly, 2017; Joiner, 2016), the core ancestral function that was responsible for the evolutionary appearance of sleep is still unknown.

What do we know about sleep patterns in ancestral pre-industrial humans? This is a difficult question since behavioral traits such as sleep do not leave a fossil record. Yetish et al., (2015) approached this question by measuring sleep patterns (duration, timing and relation to natural light and seasons) in three surviving pre-industrial societies. The three groups used were; Hazda in northern Tanzania, Kalahari San in Southern Africa and Tsimane in Bolivia. In these three populations, electricity and associated lighting and entertainment distractions were absent. These populations did not have electricity, generators or battery powered devices. The technique used by these investigators to measure sleep behaviors was a wrist worn device to monitor body activity and inactivity. These measurements could not distinguish REM and non REM forms of sleep.

The sleep period duration, defined as the interval between sleep onset and offset, was 6.9 to 8.5 hours. The sleep time, defined as the sleep period minus waking after sleep onset, was between 5.7 and 7.1 hours. Sleep efficiency, (sleep time divided by "bed" time) was between 81% and 86%. Sleep onset time occurred several hours (mean 3.3 hours) after sunset and offset time occurred before sunrise (mean one hour). Sleep occurred almost entirely during the dark period in these traditional societies in keeping with light being the major factor in human sleep and circadian control. Naps occurred on 7% of winter days and 22% of summer days; mean duration of summer naps was 32 minutes. Sleep duration varied by season being longer in the winter than in the summer. The seasonal variation in sleep duration was due to a later sleep onset in the summer; awakenings were similar in winter and summer. Perhaps one of the most telling observations was that neither the San nor Tsimane had a word for insomnia. In contrast, in industrial societies there is no seasonal variation with sleep and sleep typically continues well after sunrise. Yetish et al., (2015) did not find any evidence of a bimodal sleep pattern (two major intervals of sleep bridged by a period of wakefulness) which has been described in Western Europeans.

An early cultural innovation was our capacity to control exposure to light through the creation of artificial light. The effect of access to electric light on sleep behaviors was examined by de la Iglesia et al. (2015). The

Toba/Qom is an indigenous group in the Gran Chaco region of Argentina. The investigators chose two Toba/Qom communities; one community had 24 hour access to electric light while the second community had no access to electric light. Sleep activity and light exposure were measured with wrist data loggers. Additional information on sleep patterns was obtained through use of sleep diaries. For both populations, sleep duration was seasonal with a longer duration in winter than summer. The community with access to electric light had shorter sleep duration in winter (mean 56 minutes) and summer (mean 43 minutes) compared to the "no electric light access" community. The difference in sleep duration between the two communities was strictly due to later bedtimes and sleep onsets in the group with electric light access. Sleep offsets and rise times were the same in both communities. Light exposure during night-time was greater in the community with electric light access than in the other community.

What are the analogies between sleep and aging? Sleep is widespread throughout nature but has not yet been documented in all animal phyla. Aging is probably universal across the tree of life. Both aging and sleep show very diverse and complex patterns across species and both have very deep evolutionary roots. Sleep emerged prior to the evolution of a central nervous system and aging is observed in uni- and multicellular organisms. Both aging and sleep appear to subserve multiple functions. For example, aging programs such as cellular senescence and apoptosis are critical processes in tissue repair, morphogenesis and embryogenesis. However, for aging and sleep the core ancestral function responsible for the evolutionary emergence of each of these phenotypes is still unknown. For aging, I propose that the *core ancestral function* is the transfer of information/signaling and resources from aged organisms, both single and multicellular, to younger organisms, both single and multicellular, which leads to a behavioral change in the younger organisms.

In summary, aging and sleep behaviors are evolutionarily ancient phenotypes that are expressed in most (sleep) if not all (aging) animals. Both aging and sleep behaviors display diverse features across species and these two phenotypes are interconnected. In humans, at least, sleep behaviors change with advancing age. It is accepted that a species sleep behaviors are coded by its developmental program. Should not the same logic apply to aging?

Evolution of Human Aging

The human lineage originated in Africa and diverged from the common ancestor of bonobo and chimpanzee about 4.5 million years ago (Prufer et al., 2012). This common ancestor had an effective population size of about 45,000 individuals and at divergence the effective population size of the human lineage was about 10,000 individuals. The techniques that have been used to characterize the evolutionary course of hominins include examination of fossil finds and cultural artefacts and more recently the sequencing of ancient genomes extracted from fossils.

Two models have been proposed to account for the evolution of Homo sapiens with these differing primarily as to whether our species originated in a single region of Africa or in multiple regions (Wong, 2018; Scerri et al., 2018). Current evidence favors the multiregional explanation. Skull fossils found recently in Morocco are believed to belong to Homo sapiens and were dated to be about 315,000 years ago (Gibbons, 2017). This fossil is the oldest member of our species. It is also apparent that the morphological features of the skull that are characteristic of modern Homo sapiens did not all emerge in lockstep at the inception of our species (Wong, 2018). The appearance of a small more delicate facial structure preceded the evolution of the typical modern brain case.

The current proposal is that Homo sapiens originated in multiple regions of Africa approximately 300,000 years ago (Wong, 2018; Scerri et al., 2018). Homo sapiens were distributed in small semi-isolated populations across these many regions. These groups evolved within their own ecological niches developing their own cultures including tool use. Periodically there would be contact between the various groups which would lead to gene and cultural flow between groups. At the same time there were other archaic hominin species present such as Neanderthal and Denisovan. During subsequent migrations out of Africa, Homo sapiens encountered and interbred with Neanderthal and Denisovan. At about 40,000 years ago, Denisovan and Neanderthal disappeared and Homo sapiens became the dominant hominin species.

The results of a study by Neubauer et al., (2018) are consistent with these timelines. These investigators used computed tomography to measure endocranial casts from various hominin fossils; Homo sapiens of three geological ages (200,000 to 300,000 years ago, 115,000 to 120,000 years ago and 8,000 to 36,000 years ago), Neanderthal (40,000 to 70,000 years ago) and Homo erectus (200,000 to 1,780,000 years ago). The modern human skull is characterized by a globular endocast while archaic hominins have an anterior to posterior elongated endocast. Neubauer et al., (2017) observed that unlike Neanderthal and Homo erectus which had elongated endocasts, Homo sapiens developed a typical globular modern human endocast sometime after 100,000 years ago and before 35,000 years ago. Hence, by about 35,000 years ago, the evolution of a modern brain in Homo sapiens had been completed. It is interesting that this is the same time period in which Neanderthal and Denisovan became extinct.

The evolution of Homo sapiens was accompanied by changes in the aging pattern. Caspari and Lee (2004) looked at the evolution of longevity in the human lineage. Their data set contained archaic extinct hominins (Australopithecines) (from 3 million to 1.5 million years ago), early and middle Pleistocene Homo (from 2 million to 500,000 years ago), Neanderthal (from 130,000 to 30,000 years ago) and upper Paleolithic Europeans (from 40,000 to 12,000 years ago). Age of individuals was classified categorically as young (Y) or old (O) based upon presence or absence of eruption of the third molar tooth (M3) as well as evidence of dental wear. The age of M3 eruption was considered adulthood and old was considered as double that age. Old age, in Caspari and Lee's classification, was the age at which an adult could become a grandparent. The age data were presented as the ratio of old to young (O/Y) in the populations. The O/Y ratio progressively increased from the archaic extinct hominins through to modern times indicating that a progressive increase in longevity had occurred. However, there was a very large increase in the O/Y ratio, more than a fivefold change, between early Pleistocene Homo/

Neanderthal and upper Paleolithic Europeans. Caspari and Lee (2004) concluded that there was a trend of increased survivorship of older adults throughout human evolution. However, the increase in longevity was greatest in the early modern humans of the upper Paleolithic, between 40,000 and 12,000 years ago. Adult survivorship increased dramatically late in the course of human evolution. This large increase in longevity meant that there would be a grandparent generation present in these more modern human populations. The presence of grandparents would have made possible the intergenerational transfer of resources and information within the social group. Caspari and Lee (2004) proposed, on the basis of their data, that the increased longevity of "modern" compared to ancestral humans was the result of cultural inheritance.

Gurven and Kaplan (2007) reported an extensive review of lifespan and aging patterns in pre-agricultural hunter-gatherers. These investigators amassed a data base for the mortality patterns of extant human populations living a lifestyle most similar to that of our foraging ancestors. Some of their results for the pooled data base were as follows. About 60% of children born reached the age of 15 years. Of children reaching the age of 15 years, about 60% will live to be 45 years. The mean life expectancy for those who reached 45 years was about 20 years. All populations showed a significant post-reproductive lifespan in women. In general, these populations experienced a lengthy period of prime adulthood, delayed senescence and an overall extended lifespan. The modal age of death in these extant hunter-gatherers was 72 years with a range of 68-78 years. Modal was defined as the age at which most deaths occur. Gurven and Kaplan (2007) noted that the mean mortality pattern for these forager populations was similar to that of the Swedish population in 1751.

The important findings in these hunter-gatherer populations as summarized by Gurven and Kaplan (2007) were; post-reproductive longevity was a robust feature, adult mortality rates were low from maturity (age 15 years) to age 40 years. Thereafter mortality rate increased exponentially and the modal age of death was 72 years. This general mortality pattern of foragers is similar to that of modern humans which means that this pattern was established at least 10,000 to 12,000 years ago.

A major difference between present day human populations and hunter-gatherers were the causes of death. In the hunter-gatherer populations illnesses accounted for 70% of deaths, with 20% of deaths due to violence and accidents and only 9% of deaths due to degenerative diseases. In present day populations, degenerative diseases are the predominant cause of death.

In a more recent paper, Kaplan et al., (2017) looked at the prevalence of coronary atherosclerosis in a population of forager-horticulturalists in Bolivia, the Tsimane. The investigators reported a number of physiological traits as well as the prevalence of CT determined coronary calcifications in a cross-sectional population of 705 individuals, about 50% males, spanning the age range of 40 to 94 years.

Those 75 years of age and older had a mean systolic/diastolic blood pressure of 117.1/73.1 mmHg compared to 113.1/76.4 mmHg in those aged 40-44 years. The concentrations of blood lipid fractions did not significantly vary across the age range and mean BMI was 23.7 kg/m^2 in those aged 40-44 years compared to 24.1 kg/m^2 in those 75 years of age and older. In Tsimane, 65% of those 75 years or older were free of CT determined coronary calcifications compared to a multi ethnic population from an industrial society in which only 19% of those aged 75 or older were free of CT determined coronary calcification. The Tsimane consume a diet composed of 14% protein, 14% fat and 72% carbohydrate. They are very active physically spending 4-7 hours per day farming, hunting and doing household chores. Less than 10% of daylight hours were spent in sedentary activities.

The investigators concluded that the life style of the Tsimane is protective of the development of coronary atherosclerosis even in older individuals. I would contend that this statement has put the cart before the horse. Over thousands of years Homo sapiens has evolved within natural ecosystems and the physiological makeup of the Tsimane is the natural outcome of this evolutionary process. However, within the last 15,000 years, agricultural practices, complex societies and rampant urbanization have become the principal drivers of human evolution and aging. This change in evolutionary dynamics brings me to the second paper.

Sabatine et al., (2017) conducted a double blind placebo controlled trial of a new cholesterol lowering pharmaceutical agent. This agent is a monoclonal antibody that inhibits the protein PCSK9. The investigators enrolled 27,564 individuals into the trial and half received a placebo and half the PCSK9 antibody. Most were hypertensive and had had a myocardial infarction. Most were also receiving a statin medication for control of blood cholesterol levels. The primary endpoint was a composite of cardiovascular death, myocardial infarction, stroke and hospitalization for unstable angina or coronary vascularization. The mean duration of follow-up was 2.2 years. In the placebo group (13,780) 1563 suffered a primary event compared to 1344 in the treated group (13,784). This is an absolute reduction of 1.5%. The treated group had 219 fewer primary events than the placebo group.

My point is as follows. The genome of pre-industrial hunter-gatherers (e.g., Tsimane) is not very different from that of the subjects in the trial reported by Sabatine et al., (2017). The evidence of widespread cardiovascular "disease" in these subjects is the biological cost of living in a modern industrialized and technologically-rich urban ecosystem. The human aging phenotype has changed over the past 10,000 to 15,000 years due to the influence of cultural practices and this topic will be discussed in more detail in *Chapter 3: Aging, Diseases and Culture.*

In summary, the human lineage diverged from a common ancestor with bonobo and chimpanzee about 4.5 million years ago. The earliest forms of Homo sapiens emerged about 300,000 years ago in Africa. Although still controversial, it is believed that our species developed in multiple regions of Africa and that these different groups were semi-isolated. Homo sapiens migrated out of Africa in several waves and by about 15,000 years ago had reached the four corners of the globe. During these migrations, Homo sapiens interbred with other archaic hominin species, in particular Neanderthal in Eurasia and Denisovan in eastern Asia. Modern humans carry Denisovan and Neanderthal DNA from these encounters. Over the evolutionary course of the human lineage there has been a progressive increase in longevity. However, the largest increase in longevity occurred about 40,000 years ago, the same time period, that

Homo sapiens evolved the modern human globular brain. Hence, about 40,000 years ago seems to be a pivotal period. Homo sapiens were living long enough that social groups would contain a grandparent generation with all of the advantages that having an older generation bestow. Females by this time had probably evolved a prolonged post reproductive lifespan. By 15,000 years ago, the modern pattern of human aging had been established in hunter-gatherer populations with lifespan being limited by accidents, violence and infectious illnesses.

In this section, we have primarily focused on the time period between the emergence of the human lineage 4.5 million years ago to approximately 10,000 to 15,000 years ago. Over this span the hominin population grew from about 10,000 individuals at time of divergence from our common ancestor with chimpanzee and bonobo to between one to ten million modern humans 10,000 years ago (Wikipedia). Homo sapiens arose about 300,000 years ago and our modern pattern of aging was fully established within hunter-gatherer populations 10,000 to 15,000 years ago. In *Chapter 3: Aging, Diseases and Culture* we will explore these last 10,000 to 15,000 years of human evolution. Over this time frame our population has exponentially exploded from one to ten million to about 7.7 billion individuals. Over the past 10,000 to 15,000 years our lifespan has increased but the features of our aging pattern have decidedly changed. All of this has been fueled not by the force of natural selection but by our ever evolving culture with its technological advances.

Culture evolved among archaic hominins, but it is Homo sapiens of all the hominin species that developed the most sophisticated culture. Cultural practices, including tool use, allowed Homo sapiens to spread across the globe and to outcompete other hominins such as Neanderthal and Denisovan. By about 40,000 years ago, anatomically and behaviorally modern humans had evolved. Our large sophisticated brain fueled cultural advancements. Our longevity and social groupings with a grandparent generation facilitated the passage of cultural practices between generations. When agriculture and domestication of plants and animals emerged about 10,000 to 12,000 years ago, the stage was set for urbanization and the rapid evolution of cultural practices including technological advances. Culture has now become the dominant driving force in human evolution and has changed the aging pattern that was present in human pre-industrial hunter-gatherer populations. The two studies described in a previous paragraph, one by Kaplan et al. (2017) on the Tsimane hunter-gatherers of Bolivia and the study by Sabatine et al., (2017) highlight the impact of modern culture on aging.

Culture is a special attribute that distinguishes Homo sapiens from other species and culture has allowed our species to become a dominant global agent. I will define culture as a body of knowledge and practices that is socially learned, that is modified and added to by each generation and which can be transmitted vertically from generation to generation and laterally within a generation with high fidelity. Other species have culture but a defining feature of human culture is that it is cumulative. The passage of culture between generations is referred to as cultural inheritance. I will consider the process of niche construction as a subcomponent of culture. Niche construction is the process whereby organisms actively modify their own and indirectly other's ecological niches. The passage of modified ecological niches between generations is termed ecological inheritance.

Two important questions arise from this discussion on the *Evolution of human aging*. What role did grandparents play in the evolutionary trajectory of Homo sapiens and how did human cumulative culture evolve? These two questions turn out to be interconnected.

Grandparents and Evolution of Human Cumulative Culture

Role of Grandparents

As discussed in the previous section, Caspari and Lee (2004) found that during the course of human evolution adult survivorship significantly increased recently, about 40,000 years ago. This dramatic increase in adult survivorship meant that for the first time older adults in the human population outnumbered younger adults and social groups could have a grandparent generation. The timing of this increase in longevity coincided with the full evolution of an anatomically and (presumably) cognitively modern human brain. Caspari (2016) questioned what process accounted for this recent change in human longevity and this investigator proposed that culture was the driver of this change.

The consequences of increased longevity were far reaching (Caspari, 2016). As more adults survived to an older age, a grandparent generation became established in modern human populations. Grandparents transfer resources and information to descendants thereby increasing both the number of offspring their children can have and the survival of those children. In addition, this intergenerational transfer is a critical process in the evolution of a cumulative form of culture which is special to humans. In this context emergence of a grandparent generation and evolution of human cumulative culture intersect.

In addition to humans, other long living mammals have accrued benefits from a grandparent generation. One example is the elephant, a long lived terrestrial mammal. Elephants form matrilineal family groups of mothers and offspring generally led by an elder female matriarch. Males spend most of their time alone or with other males.

Lahdenpera et al., (2014) assessed reproductive senescence in semi-captive female Asian elephants. They observed that many elephants continued to reproduce into late life even at an age of 65 years. A small percentage did have a prolonged post reproductive lifespan but most do not. Post reproductive representation in this female elephant population was 12.8% compared to a value of 42.5% for the pre-industrial Dobe!Kung previously described. Hence, although elephants can live more than 60 years, females do not have the extended post reproductive lifespan characteristic of female humans.

Lee et al., (2016) did an extensive study of wild female African elephants which included assessment of both reproductive senescence as well as the effects of a grandmother generation. Their data base included 834 individually known wild African elephants over a 40 plus year study period.

In their study population, 95% of females had died by age 65 years. Reproductive rate declined after age 40 years and 95% of females had ceased reproduction by age 49 years. This pattern differs from human populations in which cessation of reproduction reaches essentially 100% years prior to death (Alberts et al., 2013; Croft et al., 2015). The minimum breeding age was 9 years and daughters with a mother that survived for at least their first 9 years of life had a greater longevity than did daughters whose mothers died prior to their first 9 years of life. Hence maternal longevity within families improved survival of daughters to reproductive age. There were many examples of mother-daughter pairs simultaneously breeding. For this population of mother-daughter co-breeding pairs, daughters had an enhanced age-specific rate of reproduction the longer the duration in time of overlap between mother-daughter co-breeding. Only ten of 281 mothers survived for more than ten years without giving birth, while their daughters were still reproducing, indicating that exclusive grandmothering in the absence of reproduction is not an elephant trait in contrast to humans. In essence, a female can bestow the benefits of grandmothering to her kin group without necessarily being in a post reproductive state.

Lee et al., (2016) pointed out that the longevity of elephants with creation of a grandmother generation has many advantages. Elder females are repositories of knowledge and they actively grandmother calves providing protection and social cohesion while mothering their own offspring. As Lee et al., (2016) observed maternal longevity increased survival of daughters and grandmothers enhanced the reproductive rate of daughters even though the grandmothers had not ceased breeding.

These observations in elephants underscore the importance of grandparents (grandmothers in the case of elephants) in enhancing both kin and social group fitness. These observations are consistent with the proposal that as human longevity increased and a long post reproductive lifespan in females evolved, grandparents became important instruments of kin fitness and cultural evolution.

Cumulative Culture

What about the second question; how did human cumulative culture evolve? This question intersects with another question; what accounts for the evolution of the cognitively sophisticated human brain? Answers to this latter question have fallen into two broad categories. One account proposed that the emergence of cumulative culture was the primary event and became the driver of human brain evolution. In this account, as culture evolved and became more complex, humans required a brain that would allow them to function within this evolving complicated social context. The other category proposed that evolution of a cognitively sophisticated human brain was the primary event which secondarily made possible the development of our distinctive cumulative culture. Can we distinguish between these two broad categories?

Laland (2018) reviewed this area of brain-culture coevolution and has proposed that culture was the primary process that drove the evolution of our large brain, intelligence and language. Social learning is the foundational process underlying culture. The simplest definition of social learning is learning by observation or interaction with another animal, usually a conspecific. The result of this observation/interaction is that the learner animal copies or imitates the action of the other animal.

One example of social learning by animals is that of tool use for food gathering by different populations of chimpanzees (Laland, 2018). Foraging practices among different groups of chimpanzees include cracking open nuts with a stone hammer or fishing for ants with a stick and the young in these groups learn these practices by copying more experienced individuals.

A second example of social learning involves the migration of ungulates. Ungulate migration, which can span more than 1,000 km, is an adaptive behavior which allows these animals to maximize food intake and quality by synchronizing their movements with the emergence of high quality plants along the migratory corridor. The migratory pathway is not just determined by origin and destination but also by the ability of ungulates to track the timing of spring green-up along specific corridors.

This behavior, known as "green-wave surfing" allows the animals to keep pace with the spring timing of plant greening along the migratory corridor and thus get access to the highest quality of forage while migrating, when plants are first greening up. Jesmer et al., (2018) used a natural experiment involving two ungulate species, bighorn sheep and moose, to test whether migration of bighorn sheep and moose was a socially learned, culturally transmitted behavior.

Across the American west many bighorn ship were extirpated in the late 1800s through hunting and transmission of disease from domestic sheep. Subsequently, conservation efforts were directed at restoring these lost populations by translocating animals from other populations into these vacant landscapes. These animals had no knowledge about the landscapes into which they were translocated. The investigators compared the migratory behavior of 80 translocated bighorn sheep with 129 bighorn sheep sampled from four populations that had resided in the same location for more than 200 years; "historical control group". Migration was monitored using GPS collars. Migration was defined as movement between distinct seasonal ranges with green-wave surfing along the migratory pathway. Within the control group, 65 to 100% of individuals migrated while only seven of the translocated sheep migrated and these seven had been translocated into an existing population. The observation that sheep translocated into a novel landscape where they had no prior experience did not migrate is consistent with the concept that migration is a socially leaned and culturally transmitted behavior.

Jesmer et al., (2018) developed a metric to measure green-surfing knowledge and using this metric they compared the green-surfing "knowledge" of the control and translocated group. They found that historical control populations had about twice as much the green-surfing knowledge as the translocated group. To measure the role of vertical transmission of green-surfing knowledge across generations, they used additional populations. These included 58 additional bighorn sheep and four moose populations; these groups had been translocated or underwent natural colonization between 10 to 110 years previously. Surfing knowledge for both species gradually increased with time since population establishment. They found that as the surfing knowledge of animals increased so did their propensity to migrate (percentage of animals migrating) and that it took many generations for migration to be established in animals after colonizing or being transplanted into a new landscape.

Jesmer et al., (2018) proposed the following sequence of events. Ungulates acquire knowledge of local plant phenological patterns through social learning and vertical cultural transmission across generations. After translocation to a novel region, the population begins to acquire and accumulate local plant phenological knowledge. Such knowledge is essential for green-surfing. This knowledge is socially learned within the population and passed down to subsequent generations with each generation adding to the knowledge it transmits to the next generation. This ratcheting effect applied over many generations leads to full migration of that population. Ungulate migration represents an example of a socially learned culturally transmitted behavior.

These and other examples (Laland, 2018) indicate that social learning of behaviors is a common process across species. Since, social learning is the foundational step in the creation of culture, it is clear that many species will have culture, although not as sophisticated a form as that of modern humans. Since social learning is an adaptive behavior, it will act to select out changes in brain organization and structure that promote and enhance this behavior. This proposal leads to the prediction that social learning (and allied behaviors) should positively correlate with the process of encephalization. Reader and Laland (2002) tested this prediction in non-human primates.

These investigators used the published literature to assess the frequency of three behaviors, social learning, innovation and episodes of tool use across 116 species of non-human primates. They plotted the frequencies of these behaviors against what they termed the executive brain volume of these same species. Executive brain volume was defined as the sum of the volumes of neocortex and striatum and they used in their analysis both absolute values for executive brain volume and a relative value which was executive brain volume divided by brainstem volume.

Reader and Laland (2002) found a positive correlation between all three behaviors, social learning, tool use and innovation, and executive brain volume, both absolute and relative. There were also correlations between pairs of the three behaviors. These observations are consistent with the proposal that behaviors which are responsible for the creation of culture were the primary drivers in the evolution of a cognitively sophisticated brain.

Van Leeuwen et al., (2018) reported experiments in chimpanzees examining for the underpinnings of population level variation of social behaviors. The test subjects consisted of four populations of chimpanzee living in forested enclosures in Zambia. These four populations shared the same ecological environment thus controlling for ecological variables as an explanation for intraspecific variation in social behaviors. A number of social parameters, behavioral and structural, were measured. These parameters included; party size (number of individuals forming groupings), proximity (probability for any two population members to associate in close proximity defined as within one meter), grooming (the probability of any two population members to engage in grooming) and social network attributes. These attributes included a clustering coefficient (measure of group cohesiveness), modularity (measure of group fragmentation) and social differentiation (measure of variability in probability of association among pairs of individuals).

The party size was significantly different between the four study populations after controlling for population size. The tendency to organize in groupings of specific sizes was a stable population-level feature across time. Measured close proximity also differed significantly across the four populations. However, this variation in the probability of close association across populations could be explained by differences in population size i.e., in large populations there was an inability to form social bonds with all individuals. The probability of any two members to engage in grooming varied across populations and as with proximity could be accounted for by population size. In terms of social network attributes, these parameters showed substantial variation between populations independent of population size. These measurements reveal significant differences in sociality between the four study populations. Two of the populations were closely matched in demography and subspecies. The observation that these two populations showed differences in the measured parameters of sociality makes genetic differences an unlikely possibility to explain variation across populations.

The investigators concluded that these population level intraspecific variations in sociality were culturally based. Across chimpanzee populations, there were significant variations in sociality attributes such as size of grouping, pair grooming, strength of pair associations and network interactions such as group cohesion. These intraspecific variations could not be accounted for by ecological or genetic differences and hence probably reflected natural cultural variations. For any species including our own, we must not view culture as a monolithic entity. Within any given species, there will be population level variation in culture that is not rooted in ecological or genetic differences.

These observations of van Leeuwen et al., (2018) imply that specific hominin species, including Homo sapiens, would have displayed intraspecific population level variations in social learning and in culture. This construct is consistent with the hypothesis that Homo sapiens emerged at multiple sites in Africa in the form of small semi-isolated populations characterized by cultural differences. Part of these cultural differences would have been due to natural variations.

In summary, social learning of behaviors is a common process among animals and this process would have been operative in archaic hominin species after divergence of the human lineage from the common ancestor with bonobo and chimpanzee. In archaic hominins, social learning would have resulted in an early form of culture and also would have acted to select for changes in brain cognitive functions that promoted and enhanced this process of social learning. This positive feedback loop between social learning and selection for more enhanced brain functions would have resulted through a ratcheting effect in the evolution of larger and more cognitively sophisticated brains over evolutionary time. This feedback loop and ratcheting effect was amplified in Homo sapiens resulting in the emergence of a highly complex brain capable of additional functions such as teaching and creation of verbal and written symbolic language. In Homo sapiens, these behaviors of social learning, teaching and language allowed for the accurate transmission of cumulative culture between generations. However, it is important to emphasize that evolution of the modern human brain was driven primarily by the behaviors that were responsible for the creation of cumulative culture.

SPECIATION AND DEVELOPMENTAL PROGRAMS

Speciation

Background

As a species evolves, phenotypic variations arise and if they are genetically inherited they can be passed onto subsequent generations. In essence, these phenotypic variants become incorporated into the developmental program of that species, thus changing that program. This same sequence is true when a cultural practice has selected for a new phenotype. The classical example in humans was the introduction of dairying. This agricultural practice selected out for lactase persistence which then spread throughout the population (Singer, 2018 b). Prior to the introduction of dairying, rare individuals possessed the alleles responsible for persistence of an active form of the enzyme lactase into adulthood. After dairying was introduced, most members of the population would have eventually possessed these alleles. This spread of lactase persistence was equivalent to a change in the developmental program of that population. My point is that the evolution of species and the emergence of new species are in reality based upon changes in developmental programs. Under natural or cultural selection, phenotypic variations that are adaptive will be transmitted to subsequent generations provided these variations are genetically inherited. The mechanism of genetic transmission across generations is via the developmental program of the parent.

Plastic developmental programs code the morphology, suite of behaviors and aging pattern that characterize a species. During evolution of a species, selection will lead to phenotypic changes which reflect underlying inherited changes in its developmental program. When enough changes in the developmental program of a species have accumulated, a new species will emerge with its own distinct morphology, repertoire of behaviors and aging. New species arise from existing species. Hence, the key to understanding aging as a species-specific phenotype is in understanding speciation and developmental programs. However, understanding aging is just one aspect of the larger challenge of understanding how developmental programs evolve and how this relates to the process of speciation.

As in previous sections, it is important to define terms. How do we define a species? The question of "what is a species?" has been addressed by a number of investigators (Mallet, 2008; Baker and Bradley, 2006; de Queiroz, 2007). In this book a species will be defined as a population of interbreeding animals that is distinct from other interbreeding populations by virtue of relative reproductive isolation. The various conceptualizations of species differ depending upon how the boundaries between interbreeding populations are defined and measured i.e., how much reproductive isolation is necessary to define a new species. Different conceptualizations will obviously lead to different estimates as to the number of existing species.

How do we conceptualize the process of speciation? Speciation involves lineage divergence with emergence of a new interbreeding population through genetic differentiation. This new population would have distinctive phenotypic traits and a variable degree of reproductive isolation. Speciation is driven primarily by the action of natural selection with secondary involvement of hybridization and phenotypic plasticity rather than neutral processes (Singer, 2018 a; Shapiro et al., 2016; Guerrero-Bosagna, 2017). Several questions remain open. How much divergence across the genome is needed for speciation and what fraction of the genome within an individual is shaped by selection or drift (Shapiro et al., 2016)?

In a recent special issue of the journal Evolutionary Biology, Santini et al., (2012) highlighted a number of as yet controversial aspects of speciation. These aspects span the gamut from the definition of what constitutes a species to what are the barriers to reproduction between species. It is clear that there is currently no consensus as to the definition of a species and by default no current consensus as to the boundaries that delimit the process of speciation.

Some General Features of Speciation

Speciation can occur in bursts or waves characterized by an initial rapid phase of diversification in which organisms expand into new ecological niches followed by a slower phase when ecological niches become filled. This pattern of speciation is known as adaptive radiation. Generally the driver of these radiations is the evolution of adaptive heritable phenotypic traits that allow animals to take advantage of new niches. Sometimes an adaptive radiation follows a catastrophic event such as happened at the end-Cretaceous extinction.

Species occupy ecological niches which collectively form an ecosystem. The relative abundance of species within an ecosystem is a regulated parameter since the functionality of the ecosystem is dependent upon interactions between species (Singer, 2018 b). One of the mechanisms regulating species relative abundance is through the action of population density dependence. Density dependence can be direct or indirect which latter type involves a time delay. Such a time delay can occur if the density dependence is mediated by species interactions e.g., an increase in abundance of one species has a time lagged negative impact on the abundance of the interacting species (Row et al., 2014). An experimental demonstration of the action of density dependence was presented by Karels and Boonstra (2000).

The test subject for this study was the arctic ground squirrel which lives in the boreal forest in southwestern Yukon. Previous experimental manipulations of a population of this squirrel indicated that population size was regulated by an interaction between food and predators. Exclusion of predators or food addition increased population density by a factor of two to nine but predator exclusion combined with food addition increased population density by a factor of almost 20. After the previous experimental manipulations had ended, it took two years for densities of squirrels in the experimental sites to converge to those on the control sites. During these two years, Karels and Boonstra (2000) monitored the squirrel population in terms of reproduction (lactation, weaning success and litter size), emigration from the monitored area and survival including winter hibernation survival. Overall the annual rate of population change was strongly and negatively correlated with population density. Two variables predominantly accounted for this relationship; proportion of females weaning a litter and proportion of adult females surviving winter hibernation. Both of these variables were strongly and negatively correlated with population density. In fact, overwinter survival alone accounted for about 79% of the variation in annual rates of population change while both variables explained 90% of the variance.

In summary, density dependent processes are an important mechanism for regulating a species population size within the context of its ecosystem. In the study of Karels and Boonstra (2000), density dependent female reproductive behavior and density dependent overwinter survival of females were the principal components regulating annual rates of population change with overwinter survival being the more important of the two. In arctic ground squirrels, density dependent regulation effected population size by changing female reproductive success and survival, components of the aging phenotype.

The process of hybridization is an important process in speciation. Classically gene flow between populations has been considered to result in those populations becoming more similar. However, recent discoveries of gene flow through interbreeding between hominin lineages have revealed that the results are much more complex. Ackerman et al., (2016) reviewed documented hybridization events between Homo sapiens, Neanderthals and Denisovans. The latter two lineages went extinct about 40,000 years ago. Gene flow between lineages can affect separate regions of the genome and the result can be diversification and innovation. Neanderthal genes related to keratin production have affected skin and hair phenotypes in Homo sapiens. Adaptation of modern Tibetans to living at a high altitude low oxygen environment has been underwritten partially by Denisovan genes. Ackerman et al., (2016) view the process of hybridization to be so important in the evolution of modern humans that this process has actually blurred the boundaries of what have been considered separate species. Hybridization can lead to the emergence of new lineages as well as the merging of existing lineages. Within this framework, defining what constitutes Homo sapiens as a separate species becomes more nuanced and Ackerman et al., (2016) posed the question as to whether Neanderthal and Denisovan should actually be considered species separate from Homo sapiens.

Developmental Programs

What is a developmental program? There is no agreed upon definition of what constitutes a developmental program and defining this biological process is easiest done by example. Embryogenesis is considered the expression of a species-specific developmental program and one that has a genetic basis. Embryogenesis is also a plastic process; there is considerable between-individual variation in function and form at the time of birth.

Developmental programs can be approached at several levels. As described in a previous section, speciation involves the genetic differentiation of a population of interbreeding animals. The genetic distinctiveness that defines the boundaries of a species encompasses the specific developmental programs characteristic of that species. However, species-specific developmental programs are plastic and display considerable intra-specific (between individual) variation. Developmental programs can also be approached at the level of clades since developmental programs within a clade of animals share certain features. In the next sections developmental programs will be described in terms of these different hierarchal levels.

Classifying developmental programs according to different taxonomic levels is artificial, but it is a useful strategy for teasing apart underlying mechanisms. For example, the species Homo sapiens belongs to the phylum Chordata and the subphylum vertebrata. During human embryogenesis the general organizational features of a chordate/vertebrate are laid down and then a body plan specific to our species is incorporated into this phylum-specific body plan. However, this is a continuous developmental process and not necessarily separable into distinct phylum level and species level stages.

Level of Phyla

Animals belonging to the same phylum share a basic body plan (Irie and Kuratani 2014). For example all vertebrates have a dorsally located central nervous system, segmental trunk muscles, vertebrae along the anterior-posterior axis, a complex head with visual and auditory sensory organs and complex organs such as a heart and liver to name a few. This basic body plan has remained intact across evolutionary time while other features at the species level such as body mass, color and specific morphology display extreme variation. One proposal, the developmental hour glass model (Irie and Kuratani 2014) has been described to account for common phyla body plans but diverse species body plans. However, it is important to remember that ultimately the evolution of body plans at the phylum and species levels has been driven by the interactions between ecological processes, opportunities and phenotypic/genetic variation.

The hourglass model was based on the observation that morphological patterns during embryogenesis across species within a phylum diverged extensively early and late compared to the middle of the developmental process. The middle period or waist was characterized by a conserved morphology such that species within each animal phylum showed a maximum similarity at this stage of development. This model proposed that the most conserved embryonic stage of animal phyla is not the earliest fertilized egg stage but a mid-embryonic stage known as the phylotypic period (Irie and Kuratani 2014). According to this model, at the phylotypic period, the basic body plan of the phylum is established.

Initially the hourglass model was based on morphological comparisons of species within a phylum, but recently genomic data have been used to test this proposal (Prud'homme and Gompel, 2010). Kalinka et al., (2010) looked at gene expression patterns during embryonic development in six species of Drosophila (phylum Arthropoda) separated by 40 million evolutionary years. The orthologous gene data set contained 3,019 genes and expression levels were measured at two hour intervals over embryogenesis. The divergence of gene expression levels across species was measured for different developmental time points. The investigators found that temporal gene expression divergence across all orthologous genes in the dataset followed an hourglass pattern with the least divergence (maximal conservation) occurring at the phylotypic period for the phylum Arthropoda. The genes that followed an hourglass pattern were those involved in core developmental processes whereas genes involved in secondary metabolism and the immune system did not conform to such a pattern. The data of Kalinka et al. (2010) indicated that the phylotypic stage at mid-embryogenesis was characterized by strong gene expression conservation with increasing expression divergence at developmental stages before and after this phylotypic period.

In a recent paper, Levin et al., (2016) explored the extent of gene expression divergence between phyla. These investigators selected ten distantly related species each from a different phylum. For each species, Levin et al., (2016) isolated about 70 individual embryos and measured the transcriptome for each embryo across the various developmental stages. They compared orthologous gene expression between pairs of species. The data displayed an early and late conserved expression phase separated by a mid-development phase that was much less conserved. The early phase was dominated by genes involved in cellular proliferation while the late phase was enriched with genes involved in cell differentiation. The mid-embryonic period was enriched with genes involved with signaling processes such as Wnt and Notch as well as genes coding transcription factors such as homeobox genes. Levin et al., (2016) found that the mid-development transition corresponded to that phylum's phylotypic period.

Levin et al. (2016) proposed that species comparisons across phyla i.e., species occupying different phyla, showed that gene expression conservation was best described by an inverse hourglass model in which gene expression was more conserved in early and late embryogenesis while at the phylotypic period, genes involved in active signaling processes and genes coding for transcription factors showed much more expression divergence (less conservation). By contrast, the hourglass model with gene expression at the phylotypic stage highly conserved but more divergent at early and late stages was characteristic of within phylum species comparisons i.e., species occupying the same phylum.

In summary, within a phylum, species development displayed a phylotypic mid-embryonic stage in which the basic phylum body plan was laid down and which was characterized by highly conserved gene assemblies compared to early and late developmental stages. By contrast between species occupying different phyla, the phylotypic stage displayed highly divergent gene assemblies compared to early and late embryogenesis. Levin et al., (2016) defined a phylum as a collection of species whose gene expression at the phylotypic stage is highly conserved but divergent when compared to species of a different phylum.

In the early stages of embryogenesis a shared body plan, common to a set of species, is laid down. In later stages, features specific to that particular species are added. But species also have characteristic behaviors, specific aging and reproductive trajectories and as well a maximum potential lifespan. Although some behaviors are learned, the neural mechanisms must be in place to enable learning processes. Developmental programs must direct all these aspects of embryogenesis. In addition, some species such as Homo sapiens have a prolonged post-natal development stage. Human brain development is not complete until about 20 plus years of age. Since each animal has a unique genome/epigenome and since environmental factors beginning in utero impact on the developmental process, each member of a species will be a unique product of its own developmental program. We can refer to this individuality as being the result of developmental program plasticity.

This brief review of developmental programs cannot possible do justice to their complexity. For example, in placental mammals there has been the question as to why an immunologic reaction does not occur at the maternal-fetal interface i.e., where fetal and maternal cells come in contact. Recent experiments using placental and uterine decidual samples from pregnancies that had been electively terminated at between 6-14 weeks of gestation have supplied some answers to this question (Rajagopalan and Long, 2018). Single-cell RNA sequencing was performed on an array of maternal and fetal cells isolated from the placenta and the decidua and it was shown that specific interactions between sets of maternal and fetal cells lead to a state of immunological tolerance.

Behaviors

In the broadest sense behaviors can be considered functional aspects of morphologies i.e., behavior is the way in which different parts of the organism function (Bertossa, 2011). This broad definition of behaviors would include the actions of protozoa to escape from a threat, to mate and replicate and to move towards a food source and feed (Bertossa, 2011). These simple behaviors are not co-ordinated by a nervous system. On the other hand, vertebrate behaviors rely upon the structure and activity of a complex nervous system. In this case, understanding the evolution and development of behaviors is more difficult since behaviors reflect an interaction between the nervous system and the animal's environment.

Duda and Zrzavy (2013) charted the evolution of primate behaviors by reconstructing behaviors that were most likely present in common ancestors at various nodes in the primate family tree. They started with seven extant species; orangutan (Sumatran and Bornean), gorilla (two species), chimpanzee, bonobo and humans (Homo sapiens). On the basis of a literature search, the investigators selected 65 characters which included life-history, socio-ecological and behavioral traits. Ancestral states for these character traits were reconstructed using the primate phylogenetic tree and character optimization analyses. Ancestral states were derived for; the common ancestor of all seven species, the common ancestor of gorilla, humans, chimpanzee and bonobo and the common ancestor of humans, chimpanzee and bonobo.

Duda and Zrzavy (2013) found that in humans out of 65 character traits, 27 were retained from the common ancestor of all seven species, four from the common ancestor of gorilla, humans, chimpanzee and bonobo and four from the common ancestor of humans, chimpanzee and bonobo. Examples of ancestral traits included; slow postnatal growth rate, postponing of first female reproduction, relatively short inter-birth interval and year round, non-seasonal, breeding. Thirty traits were novel to the human lineage after its divergence from the chimpanzee/bonobo limb. Examples of these unique human adaptations included; delayed onset of puberty, protracted post-reproductive female lifespan, extended lifespan, broadly omnivorous diet, unique bipedal locomotion and manufacture and use of elaborate tools.

The data of Duda and Zrzavy (2013) indicate that many human traits are quite ancient and originated in last common ancestors of primate species. Novel human traits were added onto this amalgam of ancient traits after human and chimpanzee/bonobo lineages diverged. Homo sapiens is the most derived primate species i.e., has the longest terminal branch following divergence from the common ancestor of homo and chimpanzee/bonobo.

The evolution of species character traits and species developmental programs share common features. Species-specific morphologies are integrated into ancestral body plans that are a common feature of larger taxa and similarly species-specific character traits are built upon ancestral suites of character traits common to larger taxa. These features underscore the continuity of the evolutionary process with respect to the diversity of species form and function.

Developmental Timing

In the mammal when an egg is fertilized by a sperm, a single cell is formed which contains the instructions to create an individual with all the characteristics of that particular species; morphology, repertoire of behaviors, life history traits including aging pattern and maximum potential lifespan. Most research has focused on developmental programs that code species-specific morphology and much less research has focused on the development of species-specific behaviors, life history traits and maximum potential lifespan. In addition, the evidence is that complex phenotypes, for example life history traits, are underwritten by a multitude of genes each with a small effect (Callaway, 2017; Wray et al., 2018). A central question is; what are the mechanisms that direct or orchestrate developmental programs and how do these mechanisms determine the time of onset and offset of specific processes i.e., developmental timing? The timing of when specific genes are turned on or off is as important in species-specific developmental programs as which genes are turned on and off since many genes have similar functions across species. To address this question, one can examine what is known about the molecular regulation of specific developmental programs.

Barry et al. (2017) took human embryonic stem cells (ESC) and mouse epiblast stem cells (EpiS) and cultured them in defined neural differentiation medium for 3weeks (EpiS) and 6 weeks (ES). Gene expression patterns were monitored; key mouse neural regulatory genes were upregulated earlier than their human orthologs, consistent with mouse embryogenesis being a faster process than that of the human. Species specific developmental timing is maintained in vitro.

The investigators questioned whether the differentiation of human ES cells would be influenced by a mouse host environment. Enhanced green fluorescent protein (EGFP) positive human ES cells or EGFP positive mouse EpiS cells were injected intramuscularly into immunocompromised mice and teratoma differentiation was followed for either 3 weeks (mouse EpiS cells) or 6 weeks (human ES cells). Differentiating EGFP positive mouse or human cells were isolated at different times over the 3 or 6 week time periods and gene expression patterns measured. The investigators focused specifically on the expression patterns for neural genes. They compared the patterns for neural genes observed in mouse or human cells differentiating as part of a teratoma (within a mouse host) with those obtained for human ES and mouse EpiS cells undergoing neural differentiation in vitro. Neural gene expression timelines found in teratomas paralleled those observed in vitro. Hence, the developmental timing of human-specific neural gene expression observed in vitro was maintained in teratomas even though other germ layer lineages were present in the teratomas and the teratomas were formed in a mouse host.

Barry et al. (2017) compared the rate of neural differentiation in utero to the in vitro rate. They timed neural gene peaks in mouse and human in vitro and then normalized this data to comparable embryonic day equivalents for these two species. They overlaid the mouse/human correlate between gene peaks and embryonic day equivalents with the Carnegie in utero stage progression for embryonic development. The trend lines between the matched gene peaks and the Carnegie stages gave nearly identical slopes. This finding indicated that rates of differentiation in vitro and in utero are remarkable similar.

Three important points about the timing of pluripotent stem cell development come out of the observations of Barry et al. (2017). First, species-specific developmental timing is maintained in vitro. Secondly, human pluripotent stem cells maintain their developmental timing in a mouse environment and thirdly developmental timing in vitro and in utero are very similar.

The data of Barry et al. (2017) are consistent with observations reported by Harrison et al. (2017). These investigators set up an experimental system consisting of single mouse embryonic stem cells (ESC) and small clumps of mouse trophoblast stem cells (TSC) cultured in a three dimensional scaffold of Matrigel extracellular matrix. The objective was to determine whether this experimental system could recapitulate normal mouse embryogenesis. Within 96 hours embryo like structures appeared through a process of self-organization. Similar to the natural process, in the experimental system a cavity first formed in the ESC compartment followed 12 hours later by cavity formation in the TSC compartment. By 96 hours the cavities in the two departments had united to form a single pro-amniotic cavity. The investigators determined that Nodal/Activin signaling by the ESC cells was responsible for cavity formation in the TSC compartment. After formation of the single cavity, induction of mesoderm and then primordial germ cells were evident in the experimental system. Wnt signaling was critical for the induction of mesoderm and both BMP and Wnt signaling were necessary for induction of primordial germ cells.

An interesting aspect of this ex vivo experimental system is that ESCs and TSCs have the capacity to spontaneously self-organize into an embryonic structure when cultured within the context of a three dimensional extracellular matrix structure. The investigators found that in a typical culture experiment 22% of all structures contained both ESCs and TSCs and that 92.7% of structures that contained both types of cells formed a characteristic embryonic cylindrical architecture with single adjoining ESC and TSC compartments.

The developmental timing mechanisms controlling this embryogenesis “in a dish” must originate in the two founding stem cell populations, embryonic stem cells and trophoblast stem cells, and the associated cross-talk between these two populations.

Metzis et al. (2018) studied the neural differentiation of mouse pluripotent stem cells (ESCs) in vitro and in vivo. In the in vitro experiments, they described a variety of chromatin markers to define different cell states during this differentiation process and then used these same markers to examine for the same cell states in vivo. In vitro, they exposed ECSs to a number of cytokine/growth factors and observed that ECSs first differentiated into neural progenitors (NPs) which had regional characteristics. They identified populations of NPs which had positional identities along the anterior-posterior (A-P) axis; anterior (forebrain/ midbrain), hindbrain and spinal cord. The investigators repeated these experiments using NPs isolated from mouse embryos using the same chromatin marks tested in the in vitro experiments. Similar to the in vitro results, they identified NPs that had the same axial A-P positional characteristics; anterior, hindbrain and spinal cord. After acquisition of axial (A-P) identity, NPs subsequently differentiated into distinct terminal neural cells characteristic of the anterior (brain) and posterior (spinal cord) parts of the central nervous system (CNS). The investigators concluded that the following sequence of steps occurred during development of the CNS. At the epiblast stage of embryogenesis, pluripotent NPs first acquired regional A-P axial identity which step preceded neural induction and emergence of cell type characteristic of the CNS. The correspondence between the in vitro and in vivo observations of Metzis et al. (2018) indicated that the sequence of developmental timing consisted of axial position identity preceding neural identity.

In summary, the data of Barry et al. (2017), Harrison et al. (2017) and Metzis et al. (2018) indicate that developmental timing appears to be an emergent property arising from individual stem cell types and their interactions with each other and with extracellular constituents. The processes involve the capacity of stem cells to self-organize into three dimensional structures and the capacity of cells to communicate with other cells through signaling molecules (Bush, 2019) and mechanical forces. The timing of sequential developmental events is coded in the fertilized egg and is specific for each species. However, there does not appear to be an overall blueprint i.e., evolution has fashioned that each step in the developmental process gives rise to the next step. The data are consistent with a model in which each step in a developmental sequence initiates or triggers the next step. This type of step by step mechanism would account for both the plasticity and stochasticity of a species developmental program.

Developmental Plasticity

Plasticity is an important attribute of developmental programs and can be defined as the capacity of the same genotype to produce phenotypic variations depending upon inputs during the development stage (Nettle and Bateson, 2015). Developmental plasticity is not to be confused with natural developmental variations that occur across individuals of the same species. These between individual variations probably result from the inherent stochasticity of developmental programs (Oates, 2011).

Developmental plasticity has been implicated in the processes of adaptive evolution and speciation (Hartenstein and Jacobs, 2013) and therefore, understanding the mechanisms underlying this phenomenon is of considerable importance. As an example, the nematode Pristionchus pacificus shows developmental plasticity with regards to adult mouth morphology and Ragsdale et al., (2013) dissected out the molecular pathways involved in this plasticity.

In the wild, P. pacificus lives in a necromenic association with scarab beetles. On the living beetle, P. pacificus remains in an arrested dauer state. When the beetle dies it exits this dauer state, resumes development and proceeds to reproductive maturity (Werner et al., 2017). During development, P. pacificus exhibited an environmentally sensitive plasticity of its feeding structures. When developing under crowded conditions, a wide mouthed eurystomatous (Eu) structure was formed, with two teeth, which allowed adults to prey on other nematodes. Development under less crowded conditions, resulted in the formation of a narrow mouthed stenostomatous (St) structure, with one tooth, which was more suitable for a diet composed predominantly of bacteria.

Ragsdale et al., (2013) found that the developmental switch for this dimorphism in mouth morphology acted through a gene, eud-1. This gene is located on the X chromosome and encodes a sulfatase homologous to the human aryl sulfatase A. This gene was expressed in several classes of somatic and pharyngeal neurons. Development under conditions of a high density of worms was associated with an increased expression of eud-1 leading to the development of the Eu mouth form. This Eu mouth structure allowed adult P. pacificus to prey on other nematodes. Development under conditions of low density was associated with decreased expression of eud-1 and the formation of the St mouth morphology. The St mouth form was more suitable for a diet of bacteria which would be more prevalent when few worms were around. The link between nematode density and eud-1 expression involved a signaling pathway which included the hormone D7-dafachronic acid and the nuclear receptor DAF12.

In summary, an environmental cue, the degree of worm density, during development of the nematode P. pacificus specified the formation of alternate mouth forms in the adult. Under conditions of high density, a mouth form developed which enabled adults to prey on other nematodes. Under conditions of low density, a mouth form developed which was more suitable for a diet of bacteria.

Aging

How might a developmental program code the aging phenotype? This is a difficult question and one that has not been directly addressed by the research community. As discussed in a previous part of this section, research on developmental programs has been almost exclusively focused on morphogenesis and in particular various stages of embryogenesis in different species. There has been much less study of developmental programs for behaviors even though each species displays its own specific repertoire of behaviors. Aging is a very different process that involves declines in cellular, organ and whole organism functions ultimately leading to death while embryogenesis is a "creative" process resulting in the birth of an individual member of a species with its specific morphology and physiology. However, there are studies that indirectly shed light on possible links between developmental programs and aging. The next section reviews examples of such studies.

Example 1: Age-Related Gene Expression in the Mosquito Anopheles Gambiae

Wang et al., (2010) analyzed age-related gene expression in adult females of the African malarial vector Anopheles gambiae. The purpose of this study was to explore the utility of gene expression patterns in determining the chronological age of female mosquitos. Female adult A. gambiae were collected on days 1, 4, 10, 19 and 28 post pupal emergence. The lifespan of adult females can be up to a month. Since blood feeding has a major impact on mosquito gene expression, two cohorts, with and without access to blood meals, were analyzed. A total of 276 transcripts were expressed differentially with age in both cohorts and of these, 179 transcripts were regulated by age alone. These 179 transcripts were further subdivided into three groups; 54 showed an increase with age, 58 showed a decrease with age and 67 showed a variable pattern with age. Gene ontology was used to assign functions to these aging genes and the investigators highlighted five functional classes. These were; stress response genes (e.g., heat shock proteins), detoxification genes, oxidoreductase coding genes (e.g., mitochondrial genes, components of respiration and organelle function), chitin metabolism genes and signal transduction genes.

The investigators compared age-related gene expression in A. gambiae with the expression pattern of orthologous genes in Drosophila melanogaster. Ten pairs of A. gambiae and D. melanogaster orthologous genes showed an age-related increase in expression in both species, seven pairs showed decreased age-related expression in both species and four pairs showed opposite trends in age-related expression between the two species.

The original purpose of Wang et al., (2010), was to determine if age-related gene expression changes could be used to grade the chronological age of adult female mosquitos. With this purpose in mind, Wang et al.,' (2010) selected candidate genes which had the highest-fold expression changes between young and old mosquitos and which expression was not affected by blood feeding. Seven candidate genes were selected, three of which showed increased expression during aging and four decreased expression during aging. The functional role of these genes in the aging process is unknown. However, for one of these candidate genes, an orthologous gene in yeast has been documented to regulate longevity.

The observations of Wang et al., (2010) suggest that changing the expression of specific groups of genes as a function of chronological age is one mechanism by which a developmental program could determine the aging trajectory.

Example 2: Age-Related Gene Expression in Humans

In a cross sectional study, Yang et al., (2015) looked at age-related gene expression changes in seven tissues derived from about 200 post–mortem human donors. These tissues included; subcutaneous adipose tissue, tibial artery, left ventricle of the heart, lung, skeletal muscle, tibial nerve and whole blood. Across these tissues, the number of genes that were either up regulated or down regulated with chronological age varied from 183 in nerve to 3,287 in whole blood. Up and down regulated genes showed a positive or negative correlation respectively with chronological age. Functional characterization of these age-related genes revealed that the dominant categories were; mitochondrion, electron transport chain, cell death and inflammation. The first two categories were associated primarily with down regulated genes and the third and fourth categories with up regulated genes. The investigators questioned whether age-related expression changes in different tissues were coordinated. They found that tibial artery and tibial nerve tissues were strongly correlated with chronological age but not so with the other tissues. In essence, different tissues appear to age at different rates.

Yang et al., (2015) looked for a link between age-related genes and genes associated with non-infectious chronic diseases. They compiled a list of disease associated genes from genome wide association studies and genes known to be associated with Mendelian inherited diseases. They examined for overlap enrichment between up or down regulated age-related genes and disease-associated genes. For example, the down regulated aging gene signature in the lung was enriched for genes associated with chronic obstructive pulmonary disease. However, they concluded that the connections between aging and non-infectious chronic diseases were very complex. The presumed link between aging and diseases is discussed in *Chapters 2 and 3.*

Yang et al., (2015) compared age-related genes in the mouse and human. They compiled a list of 6,454 and 6,576 homologous human/mouse gene pairs in heart and lung tissues respectively. In heart tissue, for example, the 6,576 homologous pairs contained 346 age-related genes in the human heart and 18 age-related genes in mouse heart. However, there was only one common age-related gene in both human and mouse heart tissue. Similarly, there were only three common age-related genes in both mouse and human lung tissue.

Four conclusions can be drawn from the data of Yang et al., (2015). First, age-related genes can be identified in different human tissues. Secondly, tissues do not appear to age at the same rate. Thirdly, the links between age-related genes ("aging genes") and disease-associated genes are very complex and fourthly, mouse and human (two different mammalian species) have different aging genes i.e., the aging phenotype is species-specific.

Example 3: Aging and Gene Expression in the Human and Chimpanzee Brain

Fraser et al., (2005) posed two questions as the basis of their study. Was the observed age –associated pattern of gene expression in the human frontal pole (previously reported) representative of other regions of the human brain? Did the human and chimpanzee brain share similar age-related changes in gene expression? The investigators used three published gene expression data sets which included age-related data for expression changes in human frontal pole and six other human brain regions. Fraser et al., (2005) identified 841 genes that had an age-associated expression pattern in the frontal pole and classified them according to whether their expression increased or decreased with chronological age. They compared the age-associated frontal pole expression changes of these 841 genes with the age-associated expression changes of these same genes in six other brain regions. Four other regions of the cerebral cortex showed excellent agreement with the aging pattern of the frontal pole. In contrast, age-associated expression changes of the cerebellum and caudate nucleus displayed little agreement with the age-associated expression pattern of the frontal pole. They concluded that the brain appeared to have different aging patterns in the cerebellum and caudate nucleus compared to frontal pole and cerebral cortex.

The investigators compared age-associated expression changes for three regions of the chimpanzee brain (prefrontal cortex, anterior cingulate cortex and cerebellum) with the age-associated expression changes of human frontal pole. The age-associated expression pattern of the chimpanzee cortex was completely different from that of human cortex.

The investigators drew three conclusions from their observations. First, age-associated expression changes were similar throughout all regions of the human cortex tested. Secondly, the human cerebellum and caudate nucleus showed a different age-associated expression pattern than that of the cortex. Thirdly, the chimpanzee cortex displayed a reproducible age-associated expression pattern of changes, but this pattern shared no detectable similarity with the aging pattern of human cortex.

The observations of Fraser et al., (2005) complement those of Yang et al., (2015) described in Example 2. Both sets of data indicate that human tissues are a mosaic of different aging rates and that aging appears to be species-specific; mouse differs from human (Yang et al. 2015) and chimpanzee differs from human (Fraser et al. 2005).

Example 4: Age-Associated Gene Expression Changes in a Longitudinal Human Study

Harris et al., (2017) performed a longitudinal study of age-associated gene expression changes using participants from the Scottish Lothian Birth Cohort 1936. The investigators recruited and studied about 800 individuals 70 years of age and repeated the study in 400 of the same individuals at age 76 years. The study population was equally divided between males and females. Peripheral blood mononuclear cells were extracted from whole blood at ages 70 and 76 years for the generation of lymphoblastoid cell lines. Transcriptome-wide gene expression levels were measured in these cell lines.

A significant difference in expression levels was identified between ages 70 and 76 years; 874 genes showed an increase in expression and 867 genes a decrease between ages 70 and 76 years. Functional ascertainment for all of these genes (those showing increased and decreased expression) indicated that immune system and defense response were the most significant domains. Functional ascertainment restricted to genes that increased in expression between ages 70 and 76 years showed enrichment for the process of protein heterotetramerization. Functional ascertainment for genes that showed decreased expression between ages 70 and 76 years showed enrichment for defense response, inflammatory response and cytokine mediated signaling pathways.

Harris et al., (2017) examined for associations between transcriptome-wide gene expression levels at age 70 years and eleven cognitive, fitness and biochemical traits as well as mortality. Manhattan plots showed that four transcripts were associated with smoking status, current smoker versus never smoker. Five transcripts were associated with longer telomere length. No transcripts were associated with cognition, six metre walk time, grip strength, C-reactive protein levels, glycohemoglobin (HbA1C) levels or mortality.

The observations of Harris et al., (2017) are important since they were obtained using a longitudinal rather than a cross sectional study design. These investigators identified genes that increased in expression and those that decreased in expression in the same group of individuals tested between ages 70 and 76 years. The functional categories associated with these genes were quite general; immune system, defense response, inflammation and cytokine signaling pathways.

Example 5: Eye Loss in Cavefish

A recent publication by Krishnan and Rohner (2017) reviewed the mechanisms underlying eye loss in cavefish. One of the best studied models is the Mexican cavefish, Astyanax mexicanus which inhabits twenty nine known caves. Surface subspecies inhabit surrounding river systems and serve as proxies for the ancestral forms. Interestingly, cavefish develop eyes similar to those of surface subspecies for the first few hours of embryogenesis. At that time eye development is arrested and a program of morphological degeneration is initiated. The first event is apoptosis of the lens which acts as a trigger for subsequent retinal degeneration and loss of the eye structure. Signaling pathways involved in normal eye development include the morphogen sonic hedgehog (SHH) and homeobox genes Pax 6, Pax 2 and Vax 1. The level of SHH along the midline of the neural plate controls the expression of Pax 6, Pax 2 and Vax 1. In cavefish subspecies, SHH levels along the midline are significantly increased thereby altering the balance of Pax 6, Pax 2 and Vax 1 expression. In addition, the evidence indicated that this regressive loss of eyes in cave fish is an adaptive phenotype driven by natural selection (Krishnan and Rohner, 2017; Rohner et al., 2013).

The genetic basis of eye regression in the cavefish is highly complex (Krishnan and Rohner, 2017). Quantitative trait loci (QTL) mapping has identified up to 48 DNA regions associated with the eye loss phenotype. One of these QTLs is near the Pax 6 gene locus. However, the specific genes in these QTLs that are responsible for cavefish eye regression have not yet been identified. In addition there is evidence that underlying cryptic (standing) genetic variation may be the evolutionary driver of eye loss in cavefish (Krishnan and Rohner, 2017; Rohner et al., 2013).

There is evidence that the heat shock protein HSP 90 can "buffer" underlying cryptic genetic variation. HSP 90 acts as a chaperone protein assisting in the folding and stability of other proteins, many of which are key signaling factors. It has been proposed that this action of HSP 90 protects organisms from the unwanted phenotypic effects of genetic polymorphisms of critical proteins i.e., HSP 90 maintains the stability of functionally correct forms of metastable proteins (Rohner et al., 2013). These investigators treated embryonic surface fish with an inhibitor of HSP 90 and observed an unusually large variation in eye size in the mature fish. HSP inhibition unmasked cryptic variation in eye size. When embryonic cavefish were treated with an HSP 90 inhibitor, there was no increase in eye size variation in mature fish suggesting that in cavefish subspecies the "genetic variation" had been already selected out.

Surface fish and cavefish are interfertile. An F2 population of crossed surface/cavefish treated with an HSP 90 inhibitor during embryogenesis showed a large variation in eye size (very large to very small) compared to variation in eye size in an untreated F2 crossed population. HSP 90 inhibition unmasked cryptic variation in eye size.

The investigators treated embryonic surface fish with an HSP 90 inhibitor then selected for offspring with the smallest eye size. They bred these small eye sized offspring and the F2 population raised in the absence of the inhibitor all displayed eye sizes at the very low end of the variation range suggesting that HSP 90 inhibition had selected out small eye size genetic variants. Once these small eye size variants were selected they could be maintained in the absence of inhibitor.

The investigators interpreted their results as follows. Ancestral surface fish possessed cryptic genetic variants for eye size that were masked by the action of HSP 90. This chaperone protein maintained the stability of polymorphic forms of critical proteins involved in eye development thus preventing unwanted phenotypes. The extreme environment of a cave habitat over stressed the HSP 90 genetic buffer mechanism, unmasking these protein genetic variants leading to selection for small eye size. This selection process was adaptive and not simply the unmasking of neutral genetic (drift) variants.

Programmed loss of eyes in cavefish can serve as a mechanistic model of the aging process. Eyes begin to develop in cavefish but early on in embryogenesis development is arrested. The early stage eye structures undergo degeneration (aging) and loss (death). Eye loss in the cavefish is an adaptive phenotype that evolved under the action of positive selection. Eye regression results in considerable energy savings; the optic tectum and eyes consume about 15% of resting metabolism and eyes have no utility for fish inhabiting a dark environment (Krishnan and Rohner, 2017). The genetic basis of the eye loss is complex and polygenic in nature; there are no specific "eye loss" genes that control this trait regression program. What are the analogies to aging? Aging is an adaptive phenotype that evolved under the action of multilevel selection Singer, 2016). Aging is controlled by species-specific developmental programs and is underwritten by many genes. There are no specific "aging" genes that control this developmental program. Eye loss is a plastic process with its plasticity due to underlying cryptic genetic variation and aging is also a plastic process.

Of course, aging leads to the death of a whole organism whereas eye loss in the cavefish is only the loss of an organ. However, the cavefish model demonstrates that a developmental program that initially directs creation of an organ can be timed intrinsically to subsequently "turn off" and "reverse course" leading to aging and death of that same organ.

Example 6: Lifecycle of the Mammalian Placenta

Cytotrophoblasts which are derived from trophoblasts fuse to form a multinucleated layer, the syncytiotrophoblast (STB), which covers the placental villi. This fusion process is mediated by syncytin genes, particularly syncytin-1 and 2 (Goldman-Wohl and Yagel, 2014). Cell fusion allows for the rapid and extensive expansion of the STB which occurs between 12 weeks and term during human pregnancy (Goldman-Wohl and Yagel, 2014). Cell fusion is also known to induce a state of cellular senescence and in keeping with this observation markers of cell senescence have been noted in the syncytiotrophoblast (Goldman-Wohl and Yagel, 2014). Fusion-induced senescence of the STB is a physiological process and one function is to prevent cell cycle progression and cell division within this complex syncytial structure (Cox and Redman, 2017). Senescent cells are characterized by a senescence associated secretory phenotype (SASP) which involves the expression and secretion of a number of cytokines, chemokines, pro-inflammatory factors and metalloproteases. It has been suggested that some of these secreted factors are involved in the timing of labor (Cox and Redman, 2017).

Menon et al., (2016) examined the role of placental cell senescence in the induction of labor. They compared placental tissues from women undergoing elective caesarean sections, term but not in labor (TNIL), with placental tissues obtained from women undergoing uncomplicated vaginal deliveries, term in labor (TL). TL placentas showed both a greater number of senescent cells in the chorion and amnion and a greater upregulation of SASP gene expression compared to TNIL placentas. The high mobility group box 1 protein (HMGB1) is released from senescent cells and this protein is involved in regulation of SASP secretion. Menon et al., (2106) found higher levels of HMGB1 in cytoplasmic fractions of TL compared to TNIL placental tissues. The investigators also found that HMGB1 increased the expression of the gene Cox-2 in the myometrium; this gene is involved in induction of labor. The investigators concluded that the secretory phenotype of placental senescence cells played a critical role in the induction of labor.

The placenta has a limited life span, about 9 months in humans, and has a life cycle that includes aging and death. Aging in this organ is adaptive; this process allows for rapid expansion of the syncytiotrophoblast and factors secreted by placental senescent cells function as signals in the induction of parturition. Aging of the placenta and aging (and loss) of eye structures in the cavefish (Example 5) are examples of the beneficial roles that aging of organs play within the context of the whole animal as a community of its interacting parts. By analogy, animal aging and death are beneficial within the context of a whole ecosystem community which is composed of a diverse mixture of interacting species.

Example 7: Reprogramming the Aging Phenotype

In 2006, Shinya Yamanaka described how four transcription factors, Oct3/4, Sox 2, Klf4 and c-Myc could reprogram adult mouse cells into embryonic-like pluripotent stem cells i.e., induced pluripotent stem cells (iPSCs) (Takahashi and Yamanaka, 2006). Although iPSCs are widely used in biological research, the molecular details of the reprograming process are still unknown.

Ocampo et al., (2016) used reprograming in a mouse aging model to determine if some of the features of the aging phenotype could be reversed. The mouse model used has a mutation in the gene Lmna and this mouse model shows signs of premature aging. A mutation in the Lmna gene is responsible for the human aging phenotype, Hutchinson-Gilford Progeria Syndrome (HGPS). The mouse model displayed a reduced lifespan, weight loss and premature aging of multiple organs. To prevent tumor formation and to prevent loss of cell identities, the investigators used "partial" reprograming. The four factors used were Oct 4, Sox2, Klf4 and c-Myc (OKSM). They created a transgenic (HGPS) mouse containing the Lmna mutation and carrying an OKSM polycystronic cassette and activator. Expression of the Yamanaka factors could be induced with doxycycline treatment. Induction of OKSM expression was done cyclically in the mouse model beginning at 8 weeks of age. The treated mice showed an increase in median and maximal lifespan compared to untreated mice as well as reduced histological aging in multiple organs, including the cardiovascular system. Treated mice also showed normalized genomic levels of the epigenetic histone marks H3K9me3 and H4K20me3. Perhaps most interesting, the treated mice did not show any alterations in the levels of lamin A/C or progerin in any analyzed tissue.

To examine the cellular effects of reprograming, the investigators took tail tip fibroblasts from the transgenic HGPS mouse model and subjected these cells to short term OKSM reprograming with doxycycline treatment. With short term reprograming the cells did not lose their identity. Treated cells compared to untreated ones showed a reduction of DNA double stranded breaks, reduced senescence associated B-galactosidase activity and restored levels of H3K9me3 and H4K20me3, two epigenetic histone marks involved in maintenance of heterochromatin. Finally treated cells showed less evidence of abnormal nuclear envelope architecture compared to untreated cells. Defects in the structure of the nuclear envelope are one of the main manifestations of HGPS in humans.

This study by Ocampo et al., (2016) raises a number of interesting questions. Firstly, if aging is the result of cumulative biological damage then one would expect that damage to be irreversible. Yet in this transgenic HGPS mouse model, evidence of aging at the tissue, cellular and biochemical levels could be reversed by partial cell reprograming. It is important to remember that the short cyclic reprograming protocol used by the investigators did not lead to loss of cell identity i.e., the cellular reprograming protocol used did not induce creation of induced pluripotent stem cells. The results of this study are inconsistent with aging being a manifestation of irreversible biological damage. The results are more consistent with aging being based upon a developmental program which was reversed by the reprograming protocol. This reversal in a developmental program is analogous to the loss of eye structure in the cavefish (Example 5). However, in the cavefish, the reversal is from development of the eye to aging and loss of this structure i.e., the opposite direction of what occurred in the Ocampo et al. (2016) experiment.

Example 8: Neural Stem Cells and Reprogramming the Aging Phenotype

Neural stem cells have been implicated in the regulation of the aging process in mice. Zhang et al., (2017) identified in the mouse, a population of hypothalamic neural stem cells (htNSCs) that showed an age-related decrease in numbers which paralleled age-related reductions in physiological functions. Ablation of this hypothalamic region in mid-age, generated mice with accelerated aging (decreased muscle endurance, coordination, treadmill performance, sociality and novel object recognition) compared to control animals. In a reverse experiment, when htNSCs from newborn mice were implanted into mid-age mice, the recipients showed prolonged survival and an improvement in age-related changes in physiological functions. Zhang et al., (2017) identified vesicles containing miRNAs within the htNSCs that were secreted as exosomes. Exosomal miRNAs were measured in CSF and their concentrations were reduced in mid-aged compared to young mice. Secreted exosomes were obtained from newborn cultured htNSCs, purified and then injected into the hypothalamic third ventricle of mid-aged mice which had undergone hypothalamic ablation. Treatment of these mice with newborn exosomal miRNAs ameliorated many of the age-related changes induced by hypothalamic ablation. Finally, injection of newborn exosomal miRNAs into the hypothalamic third ventricle of mid-aged mice improved age-related physiological changes compared to mid-aged mice injected with vehicle only.

The experimental observations of Zhang et al., (2017) complement the findings of Ocampo et al., (2016) described in *Example 7*. In the aged mouse, reprogramming differentiated cells or centrally administering exosomal miRNAs derived from newborn hypothalamic neural stem cells reverses or ameliorates age-related physiological changes. These experimental results are not supportive of a model in which aging reflects the stochastic accumulation of biological damage; they are more consistent with a model in which aging is based upon a pre-determined genetic developmental program.

Example 9: Maternal Care and Stress Responsiveness of Offspring

Developmental programs are plastic and can be modified by environmental factors. One such factor is parental care and the rat has served as a model for examining the role of maternal care in shaping offspring physiology and behaviors. Champagne et al., (2003) looked at maternal behaviors of lactating adult female rats towards their newly born pups over the first 6-8 days postpartum. The primary behaviors monitored were maternal licking and grooming as well as nursing in an arched back posture (LG-ABN). Mother-pup interactions were observed and for each mother a score was calculated as the percentage of the total number of observations (over the entire observation period) in which that mother was engaged in LG-ABN behavior. The percentage frequency distribution of LG-ABN behavior for the entire sample showed a normal distribution with a mean of 10.6% and a range of 4.9 to 19.7% i.e., for the entire sample the "average" mother did LG-ABN behavior in 10.6% of the total number of observations. The normal distribution indicates that within a population of female rats there is natural variation in LG-ABN behaviors. The investigators selected populations of High and Low LG-ABN mothers defined as animals whose percentage scores were one standard deviation above (High) or below (Low) the mean. The quantitative differences in the LG-ABN behavior of these two populations, High and Low, remained very distinct for days 3-8 postpartum, but converged after that time period. The growth and survival of offspring of High LG-ABN and Low LG-ABN mothers did not differ suggesting that this particular maternal behavior did not affect reproductive success.

Differences in maternal LG-ABN behavior over the first 6-8 days postpartum had significant effects on offspring physiology and behaviors. As adults, female offspring of High LG-ABN mothers exhibited significantly higher levels of LG-ABN maternal behavior than the adult female offspring of Low LG-ABN mothers. Cross –fostering experiments indicated that this transmission of LG-ABN behavior from mother to offspring was through a behavioral mode (social learning?) and not through a defined genetic mechanism.

Differences in maternal LG-ABN behavior were also associated with modifications in the stress response of adult offspring. Adult offspring of High LG-ABN mothers showed reduced plasma adrenocorticotropin hormone (ACTH) and corticosterone responses to acute stress compared to adult offspring of Low LG-ABN mothers (Meaney and Szyf, 2005). The mechanism underlying this effect of maternal behavior on offspring stress responsiveness was epigenetically based.

In response to stress, corticotropin releasing factor (CRF) is released from the hypothalamus. CRF regulates the synthesis and release of adrenocorticotropic hormone (ACTH) from the pituitary. ACTH in turn stimulates release of glucocorticoids from the adrenal gland. This whole pathway has a negative feedback loop mediated by glucocorticoid binding to glucocorticoid receptors in several brain regions including the hippocampus (Meaney and Szyf, 2005). Weaver et al., (2007) examined in the rat model the links between maternal LG-ABN behavior and the stress responsiveness of offspring.

Over the first week of life, offspring of High LG-ABN mothers undergo demethylation of a transcription factor response element located in the promoter region of the glucocorticoid receptor gene in the hippocampus. This site remains methylated in offspring of Low LG-ABN mothers. Demethylation of the response element resulted in increased transcription factor binding, increased expression of the glucocorticoid receptor gene and increased density of glucocorticoid receptors in the hippocampus. This increased density of hippocampal glucocorticoid receptors was associated with enhanced glucocorticoid negative feedback sensitivity, decreased hypothalamic CRF and more modest hypothalamic-pituitary-adrenal axis stress responses. Even though these epigenetic changes occurred during the first week of life, the reduced stress responsiveness of offspring of High LG-ABN mothers persisted into adulthood. These experimental observations highlight how the nature of early life maternal care can modify the developmental program of an offspring and that these modifications can persist into adulthood i.e., developmental programs are plastic.

The rat mother-pup studies echo the observations reported by Nelson et al., (2014) on institutionalized children in Romania. During the regime of Ceausescu in Romania thousands of children were institutionalized. In 2000 the Bucharest Early Intervention Project (BEIP) was launched. In this project, 136 children of age range 6 to 31 months were recruited from institutions within the Bucharest region. These children lived in a structured socially deprived environment with approximately one adult to oversee the care of 12 to 15 children. Half of these children were randomized to remain in institutional care while the other half were randomly assigned to foster care, the "intervention". A third group consisted of 72 children who were living with their biological parents and had never experienced institutional care.

The investigators noted that children in the institutional arm of the study showed greatly diminished cognitive functioning and diminished language skills whereas children in the foster care arm showed significant gains in both cognitive functioning and language skills compared to the children who remained institutionalized. There appeared to be a time sensitive window within the first 24 months of life within which foster care exerted a maximum effect on cognitive and language development.

Although fostered children had better cognitive functioning and language skills then institutionalized children, they did not perform as well as children living with their biological parents.

Institutionalized children also showed impaired physical growth (height and weight) and displayed stereotypical behaviors. Foster care improved physical development and reduced stereotypical behaviors but there was a time sensitive window within the first 12 months of life within which foster care had its maximum effect on both physical growth and stereotypical behaviors.

The results of the BEIP showed that institutionalized children who were socially deprived in early life showed multiple developmental abnormalities. These abnormalities were greatly improved by foster care provided this foster care was put in place within a defined time window.

The rat mother-pup and BEIP studies underscore the plastic nature of developmental programs (developmental plasticity) and the profound and lasting influence that parental inputs at critical time points can have on phenotypic outcomes.

Example 10: Genomic Studies in Long Living Tortoises

In a recent paper, Quesada et al., (2018) reported the genomic sequencing of two long lived tortoises; the last representative of Chelonoidis abingdonii (Galapagos Islands) and Aldabrachelys gigantea (Aldabra Atoll, Indian Ocean). These giant tortoises manifest a slow pace of aging and a lifespan in excess of 100 years. The purpose of the study was to identify potential candidate genes that might underlie the longevity and negligible senescence of these two species. Some of the reported observations were as follows. The investigators looked at 891 genes involved in immune function and found that many of these genes had duplications. For example, both tortoise species had 12 copies of the gene PRF1 which codes the protein perforin. Duplications were also identified in oncogenes and tumor suppressor genes, perhaps related to the cancer resistance of these tortoises. With respect to "aging" genes, they found duplications in genes associated with maintenance of genomic integrity and DNA repair mechanisms. Duplications were detected in the elongation factor gene EEF1A1 which is involved in protein synthesis. These gene duplications appear to be much more prominent in these long lived tortoises than in other species.

How do we interpret this type of genomic study? Natural selection acts on phenotypic variations within a species inhabiting a specific ecological niche and ecosystem. For example, the naked mole rat is a rodent species characterized by extreme longevity and negligible senescence compared to other rodents. As discussed in *Chapter 1*, these phenotypes can be accounted for by its being eusocial and fossorial. Genomic variants in the naked mole rat are merely the genetic underpinnings of its longevity and negligible senescence but the driver of these phenotypes was primarily the evolution of this species as both fossorial and eusocial. The same argument holds true for these two species of giant tortoise. The genomic variants i.e., duplications, identified by Quesada et al., (2018) are simply the genetic underpinnings of the longevity and negligible senescence of these tortoises. The evolution of their longevity and negligible senescence can only be understood within the ecological context in which these tortoises evolved. In the case of these two species, the evolutionary process resulted in developmental programs which contained extensive duplications of specific sets of genes. In other words, the aging phenotype cannot be understood through genomic studies alone.

Example 11: General Cognitive Ability in Humans

Kremen et al., (2019) performed a longitudinal study on the determinants of later life general cognitive capacity (GCC). Participants were recruited from a registry of twins serving in the United States military between 1965 and 1975. Twins were enrolled in the registry at an average age of 20 years and took the Armed Forces Qualification Test (AFQT). The AFQT is a measure of GCC and comprises seven cognitive domains derived from twenty three scores from thirteen neuropsychological tests. Participants from this registry were assessed at age 56 years (range 51 to 60 years) and again at age 62 years (range 56 to 66 years). Variables collected included; lifetime educational attainment, occupational complexity (highest level of occupation attained), engagement in cognitive-intellectual activities, physical activity and health status. The AFQT which had been taken by registrants at age 20 years was administered again at age 62 years. Participants at age 62 years also underwent MRI neuroimaging.

A number of mixed models were used to analyze the data. The analysis indicated that GCC at age 20 years was the strongest predictor of all later-life (age 62 years) cognitive measures. Age 20 years GCC accounted for 40% of the variance of age 62 years GCC and about 10% of the variance of each of the seven cognitive domains comprising the AFQT. The median percentage of variance in specific cognitive domains accounted for by lifetime education, occupational complexity and cognitive-intellectual activities was 0.77%, 0.71% and 0.45% respectively. Age 20 years GCC was significantly correlated with cortical surface area, but not mean cortical thickness, measured at age 62 years.

The investigators proposed "reverse causation" to explain their findings. Individuals with higher intellectual capacity (higher GCC) tend to attain more education, achieve higher occupational status and engage more in cognitive-intellectual activities i.e., the impact of these factors are primarily downstream of GCC.

However, the findings of this study by Kremen et al., (2019) have additional implications. It is known that the human brain undergoes prolonged postpartum maturation lasting into the early twenties of age. The finding of Kremen et al., (2019) that GCC at age 20 years explained about 40% of GCC variance at age 62 years suggests the following construct. Later-life GCC is determined by an early-life plastic developmental program. Environmental factors in middle life such as education, occupational complexity and engagement in cognitive-intellectual activities, may influence specific cognitive domains but have little impact on GCC once that early-life developmental program has been completed.

Example 12: DNA Replicative Timing and Aging

DNA replication occurs during the S-phase of the cell cycle and this replicative process occurs in a defined temporal order referred to as replication timing (RT). In mammals, DNA replication occurs in units of

400-800 kb known as replication domains (RDs). RT is closely correlated with three dimensional genome organization and gene transcription (Sima et al., 2019).

Rivera-Mulia et al., (2017) questioned the role of RT in progeroid (premature aging) phenotypes. These investigators studied RT in cells obtained from individuals with two progeroid syndromes, Hutchinson-Gilford Progeria Syndrome (HGPS) and Rothmund-Thomson Syndrome (RTS), and from healthy controls across a wide range of ages. The protocol involved measuring RT programs in progeroid and normal fibroblasts, then in fibroblasts reprogrammed back to (induced) pluripotent stem cells (iPSCs) and finally in iPSCs redifferentiated back to fibroblasts. The redifferentiation step was used as a model of disease progression. RT was measured in cells sorted into early and late S-phase.

The investigators identified a specific RT signature comprising domains that replicated in early S-phase in HGPS fibroblasts, but replicated in late S-phase in normal cells including those from naturally aged donors. The progeria-specific RT signature involved only 1.6% of the genome. Gene ontology analysis indicated that the genes in these early replicating domains in progeria fibroblasts were associated with phenotypic characteristics of HGPS. Rivera-Mulia et al., (2017) analyzed these early replicating domains for candidate genes and one gene stood out; TP63. This gene codes for transformation-related protein 63, a transcription factor which functions in developmental processes. TP63 replicated early in HGPS fibroblasts but late in fibroblasts from healthy donors across all ages. The investigators also studied fibroblasts from individuals with RTS. About 75% of the genomic domains that replicated early in HGPS fibroblasts also replicated early in RTS fibroblasts and the gene TP63 was an early replicator in both HGPS and RTS fibroblasts. In addition, the pattern of transcript isoform expression in both HGPS and RTS fibroblasts differed from that in normal fibroblasts.

When HGPS or RTS fibroblasts were reprogrammed back to iPSCs, all RT differences with normal cells were erased. However, when these RTS or HGPS iPSCs were redifferentiated back to fibroblasts, 95% of the genome replicated normally in these redifferentiated progeroid fibroblasts.

Nonetheless, upon redifferentiation, ten specific domains did reacquire the abnormal RT pattern observed in progeroid fibroblasts. The gene TP63 was within one of these ten specific domains and in these redifferentiated progeroid fibroblasts, TP63 showed both early replication and an isoform transcript pattern similar to that of progeroid fibroblasts. The investigators concluded that early RT and skewed isoform transcript expression for the gene TP63 were early events in the progeroid phenotype but they could only offer speculations as to how abnormal RT and abnormal expression of the gene TP63 were linked to the phenotypic manifestations of these two premature aging syndromes. Some of the answers to the speculations of Rivera-Mulia et al., (2017) can be found in a recent paper by Sima et al., (2019).

As noted in the previous section, RT is correlated with three dimensional genome organization. Chromatin is organized into two major compartments A and B, as well as in smaller units of self-interacting chromatin known as topologically associated domains (TADs) (Sima et al., 2019). Replicative domains (RDs) correspond to TADs whereas A/B compartments often consist of several adjacent TADs (RDs). The molecular mechanisms regulating RT are not well understood and the objective of the study by Sima et al., (2019) was to search for cis-acting DNA elements that were involved in regulation of RT. Their test system was the Dppa2/4 domain on chromosome 16 in mouse embryonic stem cells (mESCs). This domain contains three active genes; Dppa4, Dppa2 and Morc 1/Morc. These genes are essential for embryogenesis. Dppa 2 and Dppa 4 are important for maintaining a pluripotent state and Morc 1 is highly expressed in embryonic stem cells. The Dppa 2/4 domain corresponds to a TAD and is flanked on both sides by lamina-associated domains. RT of this domain shifts from early to late S-phase during loss of cell pluripotency and this event coincides with repression of all three genes, spatial compaction of the RD (TAD), movement of the domain to the nuclear periphery and a change in A/B compartment occupancy. Sima et al., (2019) identified three genomic sites within the Dppa 2/4 domain which they collectively termed early replication control elements (ERCEs). These sites were enriched in active epigenetic marks that are the hallmarks of enhancers. Deletion of all three sites caused a complete switch from early to late replication, a domain wide shift from A to B compartments, a weakening of TAD boundaries and repression of gene transcription throughout the domain. In summary, ERCEs are responsible for A/B compartmentalization, TAD architecture, gene transcription and RT of a chromosome domain. These properties of ESCEs are highly correlated but not necessarily causally linked. It remains unclear which of these changes in genome expression and organization are primary functions of ERCEs and which are secondary effects. Sima et al., (2019) predicted the existence of 1,835 putative ERCEs genome-wide in mouse embryonic stem cells.

The temporal order of DNA replication (replicative timing; RT) is highly coupled to three dimensional genome organization and gene transcription. Rivera-Mulia et al., (2017) showed that fibroblasts from individuals with a premature aging (progeroid) syndrome displayed domains with a specific early S-phase replication that differed from that of the same domains in normal fibroblasts. This specific RT signature involved 1.6% of the genome. The gene TP 63 was the strongest candidate gene within the affected replicating domains and this gene showed not only early replication but also skewed transcript isoform expression in progeroid fibroblasts. TP 63 is involved in developmental processes. Gene otology indicated that the genes in these early replicating domains were associated with phenotypic characteristics of progeroid syndromes. These observations indicated that changes in RT for developmental genes were somehow linked to the premature aging phenotype. The experimental observations of Sima et al., (2019) expand on the findings of Rivera-Mulia et aL., (2017). Sima et al., (2019) identified cis-regulatory DNA elements (ERCEs) that regulated RT, genomic organization and gene transcription in mESCs. The experimental findings of these two groups highlight the complexity of developmental programs. Cis –regulatory elements (ERCEs), which have the characteristics of enhancers, regulate RT, genome organization and gene transcription and in so doing appear to play a significant role in the aging phenotype. However, there remain many questions. How do these ERCEs regulate DNA replication timing? If this is the primary effect of ERCEs, how are three dimensional genome organization and gene transcription coupled to this primary effect?

In summary, although the studies described in these Examples do not directly address the question of how the aging phenotype is coded in a developmental program, they do describe potential mechanisms. Four of the Examples describe gene expression changes which are timed to the chronological age of the organism. Genes which display differential expression changes with age are known as aging genes. The functional ascertainment of these genes reveals that they are enriched for general categories such as mitochondrion, immune response, defense response, inflammation and signaling pathways. Changes in the expression of specific groups of genes that are timed with the organism's chronological age represent a basic mechanism by which a developmental program could code the aging phenotype. In addition, the expression patterns of aging genes differ between species consistent with the species-specific nature of the aging phenotype. The other Examples give hints as to the biological correlates of such age-associated changes in gene expression.

The cavefish starts out developing eyes but then the developmental program changes course and the eyes are lost. The placenta displays a nine month life cycle including aging and death. Senescent cells play a significant role in these life cycle stages. Factors secreted by these senescent cells act as signals to induce labor which leads to birth of an offspring and death of the placenta.

The studies involving reprogramming indicate that a developmental program coding the aging phenotype can in part be reversed.

Studies in the maternal rat model reveal that developmental programs are plastic and that the nature of maternal care received by an offspring in early life can lead to modifications in that offspring's developmental program that can persist into adulthood. An early-life developmental program establishes general cognitive capacity in humans, and once established general cognitive capacity is little influenced by environmental factors.

Finally, DNA replicative timing, which is coupled to genome three dimensional organization and gene transcription, appears to be involved in establishing the aging phenotype. However, the mechanisms and pathways linking DNA replicative timing to the aging phenotype are unknown.

Conclusion

The evidence is strong that aging is a universal phenotype i.e., all organisms age. In addition, each species is characterized by its own aging pattern. These observations can be accounted for by the construct that aging is coded by species - specific developmental programs. For a given species, its developmental program determines such features as its morphology, behaviors and aging trajectory. This program is plastic and subject to modifications by the stochastic nature of molecular processes and by environmental influences. This plasticity explains the extensive between individual variation in morphology, behaviors and aging that is observed within a species. The developmental program is triggered at the time of reproduction (for example, in humans at the union of a sperm and egg) and the timing of sequential steps in this program is largely governed by a process in which each step initiates or triggers the next step. Since aging is encoded in the developmental program, it should not be viewed as a life cycle stage i.e., aging begins at conception. The evolution of a species and the emergence of a new species i.e., speciation, are associated with changes in underlying developmental programs. Changes in developmental programs will lead to changes in the aging pattern. Hence, as an existing species evolves so will its aging pattern also evolve.

The human lineage diverged from its common ancestor with chimpanzee and bonobo about 4.5 million years ago. Homo sapiens first appeared about 300,000 years ago and by about 40,000 years ago the human brain had evolved to its current state. Around this same time period there occurred a significant increase in longevity of Homo sapiens and by about 10,000 to 15,000 years ago the aging pattern of Homo sapiens had evolved. The majority of humans died of trauma, violence and infectious diseases. The minority died of old age; the concept of non-infectious diseases had not yet emerged.

Since the human lineage emerged about 4.5 million years ago, natural selection has been the primary force acting over 99% of our lineage's evolutionary history. Hominins inhabited specific ecological niches within what I will call "natural" ecosystems. Evolutionary change was driven by the interaction between hominin genetic variation and ecological factors. The latter would have included climate changes since over the past 2.5 million years, hominins have been subjected to cyclic glacial periods. However this sequence of events gradually changed as hominins developed cumulative culture. Culture made possible the extensive migrations of Homo sapiens out of Africa. However, about 10,000 to 15,000 years ago, with the introduction of domestication of plants and animals and other agricultural practices the evolutionary trajectory of Homo sapiens took a change in course. Agriculture made possible urbanization and population growth. Over the past 15,000 years our population has exponentially grown from about 5 million to 7.7 billion individuals. Culture not natural selection is now the primary evolutionary force. Cumulative culture has allowed modern humans to create our own synthetic urban ecological niches and ecosystems. Our aging pattern has also changed over this same time period. Our lifespan has significantly increased but culture has led to the emergence of a set of chronic non-infectious diseases. In the next chapter (*Chapter 2*), I will explore the disease concept and its historical roots. In *Chapter 3*, I will examine the relationship between aging, culture and diseases. In *Chapter 3*, the focus will be on the question; how did human culture give rise to chronic non-infectious diseases?

Chapter 2

DISEASES

It is difficult to define the term disease because disease conceptualization has changed extensively over the course of human history. The most important factor shaping disease conceptualization is culture. Culture varies extensively across human populations and cultural dimensions such as the population's world view, the perceived relationship between the population and the natural world and the population's scientific belief system will determine how that population views disease causation. As a framework, I will use the following somewhat arbitrary definitions. As a broad category I will use the term sickness, defined simply as a state of ill health. This definition, however, begs the question as to how do we define health. Defining health is difficult, since as discussed in the *Introduction* section of this book, there are extensive between individual variations in physiological traits and behaviors. Sickness can be broken down into two components, disease and illness (Kleinman et al., 1978). Disease is a malfunctioning or maladaptation of biological and psychophysiological processes. Illness represents an individual's personal experiences (e.g., symptoms, functioning, expectations) when suffering from a disease. In summary, disease is generally considered to represent a specific biological entity while illness reflects symptoms and dysfunction associated with a disease at the individual level.

In this chapter, I will explore the historical roots of disease conceptualization beginning with Neanderthal. I will examine disease concepts among pre-industrial indigenous populations and then look at the divergent disease models that have evolved in Western and Eastern cultures. Finally, I will review the current biomedical disease model which is the basis of modern Western medical practice.

HISTORICAL ROOTS

Neanderthal

There are archaeological findings that give insights into Neanderthal heath care provision but since Neanderthal left no oral or written records it is impossible to infer how this hominin species conceptualized disease.

Neanderthal diverged from a common ancestor with Denisovan more than 390,000 years ago (Slon et al., 2018) and inhabited Europe and Asia from the time of divergence until about 30,000 to 40,000 years ago at which time Neanderthal went extinct. Spikins et al., (2018) reviewed the Neanderthal fossil record with regard to occurrence of trauma and signs of illness and on the basis of these findings made inferences about the provision of healthcare.

Spikins et al., (2018) described one Neanderthal fossil found in a cave in Iraq, dated to 45,000 to 70,000 years ago. This male was between 35 and 50 years of age when he died and he displayed a range of debilitating impairments. These impairments included; presumed blindness or at least reduced vision in one eye from a blow to the face, atrophied right arm as a result of a fracture with incomplete healing and deformities of his leg and foot. The important point was that these injuries had been sustained long before his death and showed signs of healing. These injuries would have made it difficult for this individual to perform manual tasks and other functions within his group and yet he survived to an advanced age.

Survival would have been impossible without others in the group providing assistance to allow his injuries to heal. Spikins et al., (2018) reviewed a number of other fossil findings that added to this picture of recovery and survival following severe debilitating traumatic injuries. However, not all the health impairments were the result of trauma. Spikins et al., (2018) described a male aged 25 to 40 years of age who suffered from extensive tooth loss and severe chronic periodontal disease.

Spikins et al., (2018) made the point that survival of individuals with debilitating injuries or infectious illnesses would have required practices such as provisioning, ensuring safety, assisting mobility, maintenance of personal hygiene and in general preservation of physiological functioning. Neanderthal also appeared to engage in other types of health practices e.g., the presence of interproximal grooves in teeth implied the use of tooth picks and there is evidence for the use of ochre as an antiseptic presumably applied to wounds.

Weyrich et al. (2017) performed a genetic analysis of dental calculus from five Neanderthal fossils; two from Spain, two from Belgium and one from Italy. This genetic information was used to infer dietary behaviors and the presence of oral diseases.

Diets differed among the Neanderthal samples. Neanderthal from Belgium had a high meat diet and as well the analysis showed that these hominins also consumed mushrooms. In contrast, Neanderthal from Spain consumed a diet that was plant based but also contained mushrooms and moulded herbaceous material. The investigators concluded that Neanderthal populations across Europe used multiple subsistence strategies according to location and food availability. Interestingly, one of the fossil samples from Spain had evidence of a dental abscess and the dental calculus from this fossil contained genetic sequences corresponding to poplar which contained the natural analgesic/anti-inflammatory agent salicylic acid (the active ingredient in aspirin) and contained sequences of the natural antibiotic producing Penicillium from moulded herbaceous material. The implication of this finding was that this individual was either self-medicating or being treated by others for his dental abscess with an analgesic and an antibiotic. In general, Neanderthal dental calculus contained less potentially pathogenic gram negative bacterial species, which are associated with plaque formation and periodontal disease, than modern humans.

In addition, Neanderthal culture appears to have placed a special emphasis on care of the body after death (Spikins et al., 2018). There is evidence that at some sites, Neanderthal practiced intentional burials and in some cases grave goods appear to have been included with the remains.

In summary, the lack of an oral or written record prevents us from deducing how Neanderthal viewed the nature of diseases or how their disease conceptualization was tied to other cultural beliefs. We can infer that Neanderthal provided medical care to individuals within the group who were suffering from debilitating injuries or severe infectious illnesses. The effects of a disease on an individual would have been clearly visible to other members of the group. A disease did not simply incapacitate an individual in a mechanical sense but rather affected that individual's functional capacity and performance as a participating member of a highly inter dependent social group (Fabrega Jr., 1975).

Neanderthal also apparently saw death as a special stage of the lifecycle although we have no idea whether Neanderthal culture had developed any concept of an afterlife.

Pre-Industrial Indigenous Populations

Konso People, Southwestern Ethiopia

The Konso tribe in Southwestern Ethiopia probably arrived at its present location about 5,000 years ago and this population has maintained a predominantly pre-industrial culture. Workneh et al., (2018) carried out, over the years 2012/2013, a qualitative exploratory study of Konso perceptions and personal meanings with respect to health and illness. The methodology involved in-depth interviews, focus group discussions and direct observations.

The concept of health has a very broad meaning in Konso culture. At the level of the individual, health is not simply the absence of illness but also includes a number of positive dimensions such as proper eating, drinking and social interactions as well as engaging in community ceremonies. There are also ecological dimensions to health which include receiving enough rain during the rainy season, having good harvests and living harmoniously with the environment. Social codes and powerful words e.g., curses play roles in shaping perceptions of health and illness.

In Konso culture, diseases are believed to be caused by supernatural forces or the natural environment. Supernatural causes include the wrath of God or gods, sorcery, witches, actions of spirits and failure to observe taboos. Ancestors are linked to health and disease beliefs. Failure of the living to maintain their traditions can upset ancestors, who would then cause misfortune to non-compliant descendants. Among the more educated members of the community who had been exposed to Western ideas, diseases were associated with more natural causes such as bacteria, germs, worms and in the case of malaria mosquitos.

On the basis of their study, Workneh et al., (2018) drew a number of conclusions. Health beliefs featured a strong influence of social prohibitions and taboos (e.g., certain foods) and obeying the clan leader. However, ecological values and maintaining the integrity of the environment were also prominent influences in shaping health and disease beliefs. In Konso culture, each individual is responsible not only for him/herself, but also for the equilibrium of the community. Good health and good fortune are rewards for good behaviors including appropriate "sacrifices" to ancestors while disease and misfortune are punishment for the omission of prescribed "sacrifices". Both indigenous Konso healers and their patients attributed disease origins to the cultural, natural, social and environmental context of the sufferer.

In summary, health among the Konso is conceptualized holistically as an integral mind/body/spirit unity related to the physiological, psychological, social and cultural well-being of the individual and the community.

Trio Tribe Northeastern South America

The Trio tribes were shifting cultivators living in groups that lacked a hierarchy, a non-stratified society. They had remained largely isolated until missionary contact occurred in the 1960s. At present the Trio reside in three small villages; two in Suriname (northeastern South America) and one in nearby Brazil (Herndon et al., 2009). In Trio culture, the shaman is primarily responsible for communication with the supernatural as well administering health care. Like other indigenous populations, Trio perceive health and disease within a broad framework that does not easily fit into the Western biomedical model. Diseases can be of spiritual (e.g., cosmic) or non-spiritual in origin. For example the ingestion of certain taboo animals can diminish the health of an individual. The shaman can either incite disease through their influence on evil spirits or mediate the course and outcome of diseases of natural origin. In Trio society, shaman have specialized knowledge of medicinal plants. One survey indicated that the Trio utilized over 318 species of plants for medicinal purposes. In 2000/2001, traditional medical clinics were established in the two Trio villages in Suriname. These two clinics were autonomously operated by community recognized shamans. Herndon et al., (2009) studied the patterns e.g., number of patient visits and diagnoses, at both of these clinics between the years 2000 and 2004. Over this time period there were over 20,000 patient visits at the two clinics combined.

In the clinics, diagnoses were made on the basis of indigenous disease conditions although the investigators attempted to translate these diagnoses into comparable biomedical terminology. Translation of diagnoses between Trio indigenous medicine and those of Western biomedicine was made difficult because Trio disease concepts do not clearly distinguish between disease symptoms and processes e.g., abdominal pain versus appendicitis. Trio disease conditions generally encompass a complex of symptoms referred to by a single hallmark symptom. For example, in Trio medicine, the term “liver pain” refers to a complex of right upper quadrant abdominal pain, jaundice, weight loss and an enlarged liver. The term “liver pain” would probably translate to hepatitis in Western biomedicine. Another example is malaria, which in Western biomedicine is classified as an infectious disease, would be diagnosed as fever, its predominant symptom, in the Trio disease framework.

Seventy-five disease conditions were recorded by Trio shamans over the study period. The ten most frequently treated disease conditions were; colds/upper respiratory tract conditions, wounds, bone/joint pain, watery diarrhea, cut wounds, dysmenorrhea, furuncle, dermatomycosis, malaise/weakness and leishmaniasis. I have listed these ten in the form of biomedical diagnoses, but these biomedical diagnoses are simply best translations of Trio diagnostic categories. The investigators noted that the translation of Trio diagnostic terms into biomedical terms is not straightforward. The term "rash" could apply to any one of four Trio conditions; pruritic dermatitis, dermatomycosis, chronic inflammation or contact dermatitis (response to an irritant).

The investigators also classified 127 anatomical structures, including all major internal organs and their anatomical relationships, identified by Trio shamans. The one exception appeared to be the pancreas which was not specifically identified by Trio shamans...

Herndon et al., (2009) noted a strong degree of convergence between Trio ethnomedicine and Western biomedicine. For example, an elder shaman commented to the investigators that a Trio disease highly correlative of cervical cancer was caused by a "devil spirit from the penis". Although, the Trio population had remained largely isolated until the 1960s, it is difficult to know how much recent contact with Western influences have permeated into Trio traditional disease concepts.

In summary, the conceptualization of health and disease by indigenous Konso and Trio populations underscores the holistic framework these populations have evolved. A healthy individual is one that is in harmony with his/her community and environment. Diseases are perceived in terms of their effects on the functioning of individuals and through these individuals on the functioning of the community as a whole. Diseases are not considered as strictly biological entities divorced from their functional consequences as is the case in the Western biomedical model. In fact, in the Western biomedical model, an individual can have a disease without manifesting any symptoms. For example, an individual can be diagnosed with hypertension or coronary artery disease and still be asymptomatic. Indigenous healers work at the interface between natural and supernatural realms and have the capacity to either cause a disease or mediate the course of a disease. One of the tools used by indigenous healers has been ethnobotany and these healers, as documented for the Trio, have developed an extensive array of plant-derived medicinal products.

As an approximation I will assume that the disease concepts of indigenous populations were those that were held by humans prior to the introduction of agriculture and the subsequent process of urbanization. Over the past 5,000 years at least, there has been a divergence in disease conceptualizations between Western world and Eastern world cultures. In general, Eastern populations (e.g., India and China) have maintained a holistic approach to health and disease while Western populations (e.g., Europe and countries Europeans colonized) have developed a disease-specific biomedical model. In the East, health depends on functional harmony within the individual and disease treatment is directed at the whole individual in terms of restoring internal harmony. In the West, the emphasis is on the disease as an independent entity and treatment is directed not to the whole individual, but to the disease itself. I will explore this divergence between Eastern and Western cultures in the next sections.

Divergence of Health and Disease Concepts between Eastern and Western Cultures

Eastern Cultures

India

Ayurveda is a traditional Hindu form of medicine that had its historic roots in the Indian subcontinent about 2,500 years ago (Narayanaswamy, 1981). The foundations of Ayurveda were established by the ancient schools of Hindu philosophical teachings and the legend is that the Hindu God, Brahma, passed this holistic knowledge of healing to the sages for the well-being of mankind (Jaiswal and Williams, 2017). Ayurveda is based upon a cosmology that the universe is composed of five elements; air, water, space or ether, earth and fire (Jaiswal and Williams 2017). These five elements form the three basic humors of the human body; Vata dosha, Pitta dosha and Kapha dosha. These three humors control the basic physiological functions of the body along with five sub-doshas for each of the principal doshas. For example, Vata dosha regulates processes such as cellular transport, electrolyte balance and waste excretion. Pitta dosha regulates processes such as body temperature, hunger and thirst while Kapha dosha regulates anabolism and lubrication of joints. The human body is composed of seven tissues (tissue fluids, fat, connective tissue, bones, marrow, muscle and semen) and three waste products, feces, urine and sweat. These seven tissues work in coordination to maintain proper physiological functioning of the body. A healthy state requires balance between the three doshas and other factors known as biological fires. There are thirteen biological fires or Agni. For example an important Agni is digestive fire. This fire controls proper digestive function and provision of energy to the entire body. Any imbalance between the three doshas or with other factors such as Agni (biological fires) causes a state of disease. A state of health in Ayurveda is also determined by an individual's lifestyle and environmental conditions.

Ayurveda employs a number of strategies to correct disease states resulting from the aforementioned imbalances. These include actions to remove toxins from the body; purgation through the use of powders or pastes, forced emesis, enemas, detoxification of blood and intranasal instillation of decoctions, oils and fumes. In addition, treatments involve the administration of plant-based medicines.

The focus of Ayurveda is holistic and directed to the patient not the disease. However, unlike indigenous concepts of health and illness, the patient's social context and environment play secondary roles. According to Narayanaswamy (1981), the fundamentals of Ayurveda are considered to be essentially true across time periods. These fundamentals are based on factors (balances) within the individual and not on extrinsic influences. Human habits may change and the environment may change but according to Ayurveda, humanity remains the same. Diseases attack the human and as long as the human is very much the same as his/her ancestor the therapeutic strategies prescribed by Ayurveda, with perhaps some modifications, should be successful.

According to Jaiswal and Williams (2017) Ayurveda is still practiced today although there are now attempts to merge this traditional medical system with Western ideas. In 1995, the Government of India established a separate department for Indian systems of Medicine and Homeopathy (Patwardhan et al., 2005). These systems included Ayurveda, Yoga, Unani and Siddha.

China

Chinese medicine is considered to have originated almost 5,000 years ago (McBurney, 2012). In ancient China, a human was considered to be a small model or microcosm of the universe. Tao was defined as the continuous whole entity of the universe, in which people formed a small part. Ch'i is the essential life force found in the body which was balanced through the opposite forces of Yin and Yang. Ch'i flows through a system of channels and conduits in the body and Ch'i is responsible for activating and maintaining all of the physiological functions of the body. A disruption of this balance resulted in disease. Yin diseases were due to particular foods and habits while Yang diseases were caused by evil winds, rain, cold and heat. The goal of treatment was to restore harmony and balance within the ill individual.

The Chinese recognize five elements, wood, fire, earth, metal and water. Each of these elements is linked to a certain body organ, sense and season. The construct of the five elements connect a person to nature especially the season. The body is divided into five functional organ networks; liver, heart, spleen, lung and kidney. These networks govern particular tissues, mental faculties and physical activities. Although these organ names are similar to those used in Western medicine, the functions of one organ in traditional Chinese medicine may contain the functions of many organs in Western medicine. Disease is the result of an imbalance between an individual's inner and outer world. There are eight guiding principles used to study the imbalances in a patient's energy and these are rooted in opposites; Yin and Yang, cold and heat, deficiency and excess, and interior and exterior. In addition there are four diagnostic tools of inspection, interrogation, listening and palpation that are used to diagnose disease.

Traditional Chinese medicine has a very long history of usage of herbal remedies, with more than 730 of such remedies categorized. About 2,000 years ago, the techniques of acupuncture and moxibustion were introduced as therapeutic procedures to alter the circulation of Ch'i in order to allow the body to heal itself. Acupuncture is the process of inserting needles at acupoints which are particular sites where Ch'i is transported to the surface of the body. Moxibustion involves applying burning moxa floss or other materials to these same acupoints. These two techniques are used to restore an individual's internal balance and harmony by restoring the circulation of Ch'i.

An important consideration in the Chinese disease conceptualization is a lapse in morals, such as neglecting one's responsibilities to ancestors. Traditional Chinese healers, shamans, employ ritualistic medicine to deal with lapses in morality. Shamans address the anxiety associated with such lapses.

In present day China, traditional Chinese medicine (TCM) and Western-based Medicine are becoming integrated (Keji and Hao, 2003; McBurney, 2012). To some extent, this integration process has resulted in a dichotomy of primarily traditional practices in rural areas and mainly modern Western-based medicine in in urban areas (McBurney, 2012).

Exposure to Western ideas began in the 1600s with the arrival of missionaries (Keji and Hao, 2003). At the end of the 19th century, the "School of Digestion and assimilation of TCM and Western Medicine" was formed. In the 1900s under the direction of Mao Zedong, there was a fostering of integration between TCM and Western medicine. This fostering occurred over several stages. In the 1950s, doctors who were versed in Western-based medicine were taught TCM and in the 1960s doctors from Western countries were brought to China and taught TCM. Programs were established with the focus on the integration of TCM and

Western-based medicine and in 1970 a national conference was held to highlight the progress achieved in this integrative process. In 1997, the first world conference on integrated Western and Chinese medicine took place in Beijing.

As noted by Keji and Hao (2003), Western-based medicine focuses on disease rather than health, on pathology rather than the person and on parts rather than the whole. The holistic approach of TCM is probably better suited to treat chronic non-infectious diseases and stress related diseases that are so prevalent in modern human societies.

In summary, Eastern cultures have evolved a holistic approach to health and disease. Traditional Indian medicine and traditional Chinese medicine are based on somewhat different cosmologies but in both cases disease results from an imbalance in vital factors and functions within an individual. Treatments are directed at the whole person, not exclusively on the disease, and focus on restoring health by correcting these inner imbalances. These systems of health and disease have been very successful and are still widely practiced in the Indian subcontinent and China. Western societies have evolved a very different health and disease system which is based on the biomedical model of health and disease. In this system the focus of treatment is the disease itself and not on the whole individual. In the next sections, I will examine the evolution of Western-based medicine.

Western Cultures

Greece

In ancient Greece, approximately 2,400 to 2,600 years ago, disease conceptualization was based upon a model in which the human body had four fluids; blood, phlegm, yellow bile and black bile (Tountas, 2009). The composition of these four fluids or humors varied across individuals. These four humors were linked to a worldview based on the existence of four elements; fire, earth, water and air. This construct of body humors linked to cosmological elements bears a striking resemblance to the foundations of Ayurveda and traditional Chinese medicine. Health was maintained through harmony and balance of these four humors, again similar to the basic teachings of Ayurveda and traditional Chinese medicine. About, 2,500 years ago, the writings of Hippocrates flourished, but it has not been determined whether the writings and teachings of Hippocrates are those of a single individual or the contributions of a group of individuals (Tountas, 2009).

As reviewed by Tountas (2009), Hippocrates taught that health was achieved through an equilibrium between environmental forces (wind, temperature, water and food) and individual habits (diet, alcohol, sexual behavior, work and leisure). This interplay between external factors and personal habits determined the internal balance of the four bodily humors or fluids which in turn determined an individual's state of health. Hippocrates, in essence, attributed disease causation to natural forces rather than supernatural forces such as evil spirits or the actions of gods. This attribution of disease causation to natural rather than supernatural forces is the major distinction between the Hippocratic system of medicine and the systems of Ayurveda and Traditional Chinese medicine.

For Hippocrates, disease was a natural process and this view is best exemplified by the description of epilepsy given by Hippocrates. Prior to the time of Hippocrates, epilepsy had been considered a sacred illness with a divine origin i.e., the wrath or vengeance of an angry god or gods. In the Ayurvedic system of medicine, epilepsy was attributed to the actions of spirits and goblins which had taken possession of the afflicted human body (Tripathi et al., 2000). The following is a quote from Hippocrates posted by the Epilepsy museum of Kork Germany. "It is thus with regard to the disease called sacred: it appears to me to be in no way more divine nor more sacred than other diseases… . The brain is the cause of this affliction… . When the (surplus) phlegm (from the brain) runs down through the veins, the patient loses his speech and foams at the mouth, his hands are contracted, the eyes contorted, he becomes insensible, and in some cases the bowels are emptied… . The patient kicks with his feet… . The patient must endure all these symptoms when the cold phlegm flows into the warm blood."

About 700 years after Hippocrates, came Galen who built upon the teachings and views of Hippocrates (Subbarayappa, 2001; Nutton, 2018). Galen was born in Asia Minor, but spent a great part of his active life in Rome. He brought together the disease concepts of Hippocrates with the results of anatomical studies he had performed in different animal species such as monkeys, pigs, sheep and goats. He believed that human health required equilibrium between the four main body humors each of which was built up from the four elements; fire, earth, water and air. He believed that humoral imbalances could occur in specific organs as well as in the body as a whole. Galen perceived the body as consisting of three interconnected systems; brain and nerves (sensation and thought) heart and arteries (responsible for life giving energy) and the liver and veins (responsible for nutrition and growth). Galen also incorporated the vital spirit pneuma into his health and disease construct. Pneuma was a fundamental life force which was drawn inside into the lungs by the act of breathing and from the lungs was distributed by blood to all the vital organs, thus sustaining life within the organism. Galen's view of disease held sway and remained influential well into the mid 1500s.

In summary, the Greek view of disease relied heavily upon the concept of body fluids and their balance or equilibrium; health was a state of balance whereas disease was a state of imbalance. However, the Greeks viewed disease states as the result of natural not supernatural factors and through Galen laid the foundation of anatomical medical knowledge.

Pre-Industrial Europe

Hippocrates fostered the idea that disease causation was due to natural as opposed to supernatural factors. Galen incorporated into this Hippocratic framework, the anatomy of bodily organs based upon his dissection of various animal species. In Western Europe from the thirteenth century onward, disease conceptualization remained pluralistic until the second half of the nineteenth century. At that time the roots of the biomedical model were established when laboratory tools were introduced.

Academic medicine originated in Southern Europe between the early twelfth and early thirteenth centuries and medical schools were established in universities (Arrizabalaga, 1999). Between the thirteenth and nineteenth centuries disease causation was based upon concepts ascribed to Hippocrates and Galen. Infectious diseases were the chief cause of death during this time period and examining changing views on causation of infectious diseases mirrors views on the broader subject of death and its causes. In this pre-laboratory period a disease such as plague was diagnosed through its symptoms. The view was that the "morbid matter" associated with the plague could freely move within the body so that the disease could change location and even be transformed into another disease (Arrizabalaga, 1999). A single cause could lead to different diseases and a single disease could have multiple causes. By contrast, in the present era of laboratory medicine, plague is diagnosed through laboratory detection of a specific microbe, Yersinia pestis, in the tissues of the ill person.

A glimpse into health concepts popular during this pre-laboratory period is provided by how the relationship between old age and natural death was conceptualized. This particular conceptualization is referred to as the "lamp metaphor", a metaphor which actually dated back to Roman times (Niebyl, 1971; Arrizabalaga, 1999). In this metaphor, radical moisture (the nutritive natural essence of the organism in the Galen framework) feeds the innate heat of life, like lamp oil feeds the flame. As radical moisture dries up, the innate heat will diminish and thus the body will become cold and dry. Natural death arrives when the innate heat is extinguished by the lack of radical moisture. At conception, each individual receives a quantitatively and qualitatively variable portion of radical moisture. The quality, quantity and adequacy of combustion of one's radical moisture, will determine whether one's life will be shorter or longer. Prolonging life required living a lifestyle that preserved radical moisture from interior and exterior insults.

The London (England) Bills of Mortality (begun in 1519) represent an early modern approach to disease classification (DeLacy, 1999) and febrile illnesses i.e., infectious diseases, constituted the main cause of death. Hence, as already noted, changes in the conceptualization of infectious diseases during this period can be used as a reflection of how disease conceptualization in general evolved.

In the late 1700s, William Black, a physician, attempted to disentangle the category "fevers" into specific entities. This goal of Black represented a very early attempt to conceptualize fevers as specific entities, each directly related to a particular pathogenic substance (DeLacy, 1999). However, even in the eighteenth century Galen's health and disease system constructed from the four elements and four humors still held sway. Disease was the result of individual differences in constitution (humors) and habits; fever was the result of excess "hot" humors. Epidemics were due to corruption of the atmosphere i.e., pollution of the air. Individual constitutional differences determined who was susceptible to the polluted air. Hence, a disease was not a specific entity but a process. There were no diseases as such, just a series of diseased patients. However, during the Renaissance, there were some alternative views. Some proposed that fevers were not the result of an internal imbalance within an individual, but actually an invasion of the body by particular morbific matter that came from outside the individual; a contagion that could be transmitted from one person to another. This model could explain why a febrile disease such as plague could cause similar symptoms in individuals with different internal humoral balances.

A particularly prescient view of the contagiousness of plague was given by Girolamo Fracastoro in 1546 (DeLacy, 1999). He proposed that diseases, like plague, were transmitted by seeds which could be spread by contact between individuals and also spread by an airborne mechanism. The air served only as a medium for transmission of specific seeds of disease from a particular source; the air itself was not corrupted. For Fracastoro, the contagion itself e.g., plague was the disease and each contagious disease was the result of a specific kind of seed. However, as plague became less frequent by the end of the 1600s Fracastoro's views became more marginalized. A parallel event during the late 1600s was the visualization of microorganisms by van Leeuwenhoek using a single lens microscope.

In the early eighteenth century epidemics of smallpox and plague led to changes in disease conceptualization (DeLacy, 1999). Experiments using the technique of smallpox inoculation by Hans Sloane in 1721, demonstrated that a particular physical substance taken from one patient could cause a nearly identical disease when inoculated into a second patient. Also, it was observed that smallpox matter was specific in that it only caused smallpox and not some other contagion. In the mid 1800s, William Cullen developed a classification of infectious disease based upon the principle that a species (type) of acute disease constituted a specific group of symptoms caused by a particular species of matter and the same matter would always cause the same disease even if the symptoms varied.

In summary, by the late 1800s the germ theory was essentially the accepted model of contagion causation. The pathway had started with Fracastoro's proposed theory in 1546, van Leeuwenhoek's direct visualization of microorganisms in the late 1600s, Sloane's inoculation experiments with smallpox in 1721, the experimental work by Louis Pasteur in the 1860s and Robert Koch's development of postulates in the 1880s which were used to confirm that a specific infectious disease was caused by a particular organism. The field of bacteriology blossomed in the late 1800s during which time pathogenic bacteria were identified followed by the discovery of viruses in the 1890s. Western based medicine had entered the laboratory era and the biomedical model would become its foundation.

The divergence between Western and Eastern disease concepts and medical models is part of a broader based fundamental difference between Western and Eastern civilizations. Frankopan (2017) clearly articulated the divergent historical narrative between Western and Eastern societies. The Eurocentric Western view portrays the history of civilization as built upon a foundation of ancient Greece and Rome followed by the ascendancy of Europe through the Renaissance, Enlightenment and industrial revolution. European colonization of North America gave birth to the United States. Ignored in this narrative are the important cultural and economic contributions of Eastern civilizations such as China and India. The influence of these Eastern civilizations was transferred to the West through the societies occupying the region between the eastern Mediterranean and the Himalayas via the silk roads.

Two observations underscore the cultural differences between Western and Eastern civilizations. First, in the field of medical technology, most advances have been developed in the Western world. Some notable examples include; stethoscope (1815), first clinical use of anesthesia (1841), detection of electrical brain activity (1874), first practical electrocardiogram machine (1903), first clinical use of a cardiac pacemaker (1936), functional dialysis machine (1943), first clinical use of a heart-lung bypass machine (1953), first practical commercial ultrasound machine (1965). Science based medical technology feeds into the medical model developed by the Western world.

Secondly, during the period between the late 1400s and late 1700s (Age of Discovery), European countries sponsored a number of worldwide sailing expeditions with the purpose of developing new global commercial markets.

These observations define features of Western culture such as entrepreneurship, a global perspective and science based activities which differ fundamentally from those found in Eastern culture. These features of Western culture are much more consistent with a biomedical model that focuses on disease, defined scientifically, as the target of medical practice than a holistic form of medical practice which is based on a philosophic and empirical foundation.

As an aside, the above mentioned worldwide sailing expeditions, executed for the purpose of economic gain, had devastating consequences on both indigenous populations and the global climate (Koch et al., 2019). In the American hemisphere the indigenous population pre-European contact was estimated to be about sixty million (Koch et al., 2019). Approximately one hundred years post-European contact the hemispheric population was estimated to be 6.1 million i.e., 90% depopulation. The primary causative factor leading to this massive depopulation was the introduction of infectious diseases, brought by the Europeans, to which the indigenous populations had no immunity. These included influenza, smallpox, measles, bubonic plague and later malaria, diphtheria, typhus and cholera. Secondary causative factors were the social consequences of these epidemics such as warfare, slavery, food shortages and forced relocations. These secondary factors amplified the direct mortality effects of these epidemics. However, Koch et al., (2019) pointed out another consequence of this extreme depopulation of indigenous populations. Land use for farming drastically fell because of this depopulation. This abandonment of farm land led to secondary regrowth of forest covering over approximately fifty six million hectares of land. This forest regrowth of abandoned land led to carbon uptake (sequestration) equivalent to a decline in atmospheric CO_2 of 3.5 ppm. Koch et al., (2019) estimated that a reduction of atmospheric CO2 of 3.5 ppm would have been associated with a reduction in global surface air temperature of between 0.03 and 0.08 $^{\circ}$ C between 1577 and 1694 CE.

Present State of Western Disease Conceptualization

The London Bills of Mortality of 1701 to 1771 (DeLacy, 1999) represented a compilation of causes of mortality during that time period. What we would classify as infectious diseases constituted the predominant assigned cause of death. Chronic non-infectious diseases, so prevalent today, were hardly referenced. Within this historical context, disease conceptualization in the Western world, described in the previous section, evolved in conjunction with changes in the understanding of the pathogenesis of infectious diseases. This evolving disease model changed from one that implicated corrupted or polluted air as the causative factor to one in which specific pathogenic microorganisms produced specific infectious diseases. However, I would contend that this specific causative model does not readily translate into a similar model to explain the causation of chronic non-infectious diseases. Chronic non-infectious diseases do not have unitary causes. With this contextual background, what is the current state of disease conceptualization within the Western world?

Diseases are classified on several levels or scales. The WHO International Classification of Diseases and preeminent medical textbooks such as Harrison's Principles of Internal Medicine (Jamieson et al., 2018) classify diseases at the scale of organ systems e.g., diseases of the cardiovascular system, disorders of the respiratory system, neurologic diseases, endocrine system and metabolism etc. Each of these organ system categories contain a collection of diseases related to specific components of that organ system. In Harrison's Principles of Internal Medicine, the large scale category, respiratory system diseases is divided into smaller scale categories such as asthma, bronchiectasis, chronic obstructive pulmonary disease and interstitial lung diseases. The category of cardiovascular diseases contains the smaller scale entity atherosclerosis and the category labeled endocrinology and metabolism contains the more specific diseases of obesity, diabetes and metabolic syndrome.

In Western medicine mind and body are considered separate. In Harrison's textbook, psychiatric diseases are classified under neurologic diseases. However, the American Psychiatric Association publishes its own classification referred to as the Diagnostic and Statistical Manual of Mental Disorders (DSM).

In both Harrison's textbook and the WHO classification, infectious diseases form a separate large scale category which is further divided into smaller scale entities representing specific infectious diseases each caused by a particular microorganism.

With advancements in molecular biology, the scale of disease categories has become even smaller. There are now protein misfolding diseases and diseases of the nuclear envelope of the cell, termed laminopathies. However, these "molecular" diseases are heterogeneous collections of other diseases. For example, laminopathies include muscular dystrophy, cardiomyopathy, lipodystrophy and progeria. Protein misfolding diseases include prion diseases and neurodegenerative diseases.

With the exception of infectious diseases, none of the non-infectious chronic diseases has a specific single cause and hence none of these diseases is curable.

In summary, Western based disease conceptualization is science based but within a heterogeneous framework. At the largest scale of classification, diseases are associated with organ systems. At smaller scales, some diseases are associated with functional disorders e.g., asthma, some with morphological changes e.g., atherosclerosis and some with molecular processes e.g., protein misfolding diseases. Except for infectious diseases, no diseases are classified according to a specific cause. Between individual variations within disease categories is downplayed and in fact all individuals with the same disease label are considered to form a uniform population. This notion is based upon the great difficulty we have in defining what are ranges of "normal" for human physiological traits and behaviors. Our science based conceptualization of disease is but one dimension of our highly technological culture and our cultural beliefs include the notion that any perceived problem, medical or otherwise, has a technological fix. In two previous publications (Singer, 2013 and 2015), I argued that chronic non-infectious diseases should be considered as variations in the aging phenotype across individuals. Our current hodgepodge of disease conceptualizations is consistent with and reinforces this conclusion.

Our association of diseases with specific organ systems parallels other aspects of Western medicine such as medical education and medical practice. Our medical curriculum uses a systems based approach. Medical knowledge is divided into organ systems and for example students are taught the physiology, anatomy and diseases of the cardiovascular system in a single block. The same process is repeated for the respiratory system, the genitourinary system etc. In this system of medical education, a human is considered to be a collection of organ systems rather than an integrated functional whole. The same approach has been taken in our practice of medicine. We have created medical specialties which parallel our organ specific disease classification. We have specialist physicians trained as cardiologists, nephrologists, endocrinologists, psychiatrists etc. This structure of medical practice discourages a holistic approach to disease and illness.

The Western based biomedical model encompassing disease conceptualization, teaching and practices is the antithesis of the holistic system characteristic of traditional Eastern based systems.

CONCLUSION

Disease conceptualization has a deep evolutionary history in hominin species. The evidence indicates that Neanderthal engaged in self-medication and ministered to the health needs of individuals with severe debilitating injuries. Without a written or oral record, we can only speculate how Neanderthal viewed disease causation. Indigenous populations developed a holistic approach to diseases which could have natural or supernatural causes. Disease conceptualization was viewed within a broad context that included not only the individual but also the interaction between the individual and his/her community and environment. Indigenous populations relied on shamans for their healing powers which included the use of plant derived medicinal preparations.

Over the past 5,000 plus years, Eastern and Western cultures diverged and one dimension of that cultural divide was disease conceptualization. Eastern culture viewed disease causation and treatment from the perspective of the whole individual and his/her environment and this conceptualization was based upon an empirical and philosophical foundation. Western culture viewed disease causation and treatment as independent of the individual and his/her environment and this conceptualization was based upon scientific knowledge. Treatment is holistic in Eastern culture and disease focused in Western culture. However, more recently, the process of globalization has diminished the cultural divide between West and East and the Western conceptualization of disease has made significant inroads into Eastern culture. Evidence of the globalization of the Western biomedical model is the recent report that Chinese scientists used the CRISPR gene editing tool to alter the genome of early stage human embryos (Normile, 2018).

In this section I will exclude infectious diseases since they are caused by particular external agents i.e., microorganisms. The term disease will be used to refer to chronic non-infectious disease only. One of the dimensions of a population's culture is how that population conceptualizes disease. Such a conceptualization is important since it determines the nature of treatment for an individual suffering from disease. The Western biomedical model has gained pre-eminence globally. Within this model, a disease is the result of one or more internal pathological processes and treatment involves the correction of these pathological processes. Social context and environmental factors are generally deemed irrelevant with respect to the choice and success of treatment. However, I would contend that disease conceptualization is a cultural construct created to accommodate the extensive between individual variations that characterize the human aging trajectory.

Humans like all animals age, but defining what constitutes a "normal" human aging trajectory is extremely difficult given that no two individuals follow the same aging pathway. Within its cultural belief system, a population creates a construct as to what constitutes a state of health and what constitutes healthy aging. Deviations from this construct are conceptualized as diseases. In Western culture a scientific foundation has been incorporated into this conceptualization i.e., the biomedical model. Diseases are not diseases as conceptualized, but simply variants of the aging process. Furthermore, over the past 10,000 to 15,000 years the human aging pattern has changed. Over this time frame, two trends have occurred; so called chronic non-infectious diseases have replaced infectious diseases as the predominant cause of mortality and human cultural practices have created our modern technologically rich urban ecosystem. In the next chapter, the relationships between aging, culture and so-called chronic non-infectious diseases will be explored in more detail. The premise is that so called chronic non-infectious diseases reflect culturally induced changes in human aging.

In summary, disease is a human cultural construct that serves at least two purposes–to explain deviations from culturally defined norms of human functioning and to describe therapies to correct those deviations. Most important, the disease construct is culturally specific since it is derived from that particular population's world view and cosmology.

Chapter 3

AGING, DISEASES AND CULTURE

Note: In this chapter I will still use the words "disease" and "chronic non-infectious disease" for the sake of simplicity even though as discussed in Chapter 2, I believe that diseases are actually variants of the aging phenotype.

BACKGROUND

In this chapter the focus will be on the role of culture, including niche construction, in shaping the aging trajectory of our species. During the last 10,000 to 15,000 years culture has become the primary driver of human evolution, in essence constraining the role of natural selection. This observation brings up an interesting question. Blount et al., (2018) reviewed the roles of contingency and determinism in evolution. Evolution can be considered an historical biological process and contingency refers to the occurrence of chance events that can change the path of evolution and hence its outcome. Natural selection is a deterministic process and the widespread occurrence of convergent evolution in nature has been used as an argument that under certain circumstances evolutionary outcomes are predictable i.e., determined (Blount et al., 2018). Unlike natural selection, culture is not a deterministic process. In this case the evolutionary outcomes driven by culture will be less predictable than those primarily driven by natural selection.

Human culture has resulted in the emergence of chronic non-infectious diseases which have become part of our aging pattern. In this *Chapter*, I will explore the mechanistic links between culture and variations in human phenotypes and in particular how culture is linked to chronic non-infectious disease phenotypes.

Culture Has Deep Evolutionary Roots

Culture has been documented in animals other than humans, including non-human primates and cetaceans. But culture has even deeper evolutionary roots as attested to by the existence of an elementary form of culture in fruit flies (Danchin et al., 2018). The behavioral trait measured was mate selection by female flies and the investigators defined culture according to the following criteria; 1) trait variation transmitted by social learning, 2) trait transmission occurring across age classes, 3) cultural inheritance maintained for a long enough period to permit copying, 4) phenotypic conformity in the study population and 5) generation of local traditions over an extended period.

Danchin et al., (2018) set up a test situation in which a female observer fruit fly separated by a transparent glass partition could watch a demonstrator female freely choose to mate with either a green marked male or a pink marked male. Immediately following this observational step, the observer female was allowed to choose to mate with one of two new males, one marked pink and one marked green. As a control situation, the transparent partition separating the observer fly was replaced with an opaque white paper. Female observer flies mated preferentially with new males of the same color as they saw being chosen by the demonstrator female (criterion 1).

To satisfy criterion 2, the ages of the flies were varied. In one test situation, both observer and demonstrator females were three days old and in a second test situation the demonstrator female was 14 days old and the observer female 3 days old. In both cases, the observer female preferentially selected to mate with a male of the same color as chosen by the demonstrator female.

To test for persistence of socially learned mate preference (criterion 3), observer females were subjected to five conditioning demonstrations (spaced by 15-30 minute rest periods) of females mating with males of either all green or all pink color and then 24 hours later, observer females were tested for mate preference. After 24 hours observer females preferred to mate with males of the same color they had observed mating with demonstrator females.

"Conformity" experiments demonstrated that female observers learned equally well to prefer the most commonly chosen male color, pink or green, regardless of whether that color was chosen 100% or 60% of the time by demonstrator females.

Finally, to test for persistence of mate preferences at a population level, the investigators performed a transmission chain experiment. Six females at step one observed mating between six demonstrator females and males all of the same color. These observer females were then used as the six freely choosing demonstrator females at the second step and so on; thus creating a cultural transmission chain. This experiment showed that even in a small population of six observer females, the original mate preference was transmitted over more steps than would have occurred by chance alone. This result suggested that even a small population of flies could develop a relatively long term stable tradition of mate preference.

In summary, female fruit flies have the cognitive capacity to socially learn mate preference. Socially learned mate preference was persistent for at least 24 hours and could be transmitted across multiple steps. These observations indicate that the cognitive capacity to socially learn a behavior and transmit this learned behavior over an extended series of steps is of ancient evolutionary origin.

In the next sections, I will describe examples of cultural driven changes in human phenotypes. I have classified these examples into two categories. In the first category, cultural driven phenotypic changes have been accompanied by genomic changes while in the second category genomic changes have not been associated with the cultural driven phenotypic changes.

Cultural Driven Changes in Human Phenotypes That Are Accompanied by Documented or Putative Genomic Changes

First we must define culture and the process of niche construction. In *Chapter 1,* culture was defined as a body of knowledge and practices that is socially learned, that is modified and added to by each generation and which can be transmitted with high fidelity both vertically from generation to generation and laterally within a generation. In this definition I have included the attribute cumulative although this attribute is probably unique to human culture. A cumulative culture such as ours can only emerge in a highly social and cooperative species.

The definition of niche construction is particularly broad as pointed out by Laland et al., (2016). These investigators listed three criteria to determine the presence of niche construction.

1) An organism must significantly modify environmental conditions.
2) Organism-mediated environmental modifications must influence selection pressures on a recipient organism.
3) There must be an evolutionary response in at least one recipient population caused by the environmental modification.

At least for humans, I will consider the process of niche construction to be a cultural practice. In contrast, although dam building by the beaver is an example of niche construction, it would not be considered a cultural practice of the beaver. In this chapter since the focus will be on humans, the term culture will include the process of niche construction.

Before considering specific examples of cultural driven phenotypic changes, it is useful to consider how culture is transmitted.

On an individual level, culture can be transmitted vertically between generations or horizontally within the same generation. On a population level, culture can be spread either by diffusion (cultural exchange) of a cultural practice from one population to another or by the migration of a population with its specific culture to another area. The cultural practice of dairy farming illustrates these two modes of population level cultural spread (Jeong et al., 2018, Orlando, 2018).

Based upon archaeological finds, dairy consumption appeared about 2,000 years after domestication of cattle (Orlando, 2018). Cattle specific proteins were detected in vessel remains in Turkey dating back approximately 8,000 years ago. Early evidence of dairy products has been found in various regions as follows; Europe, 6,800 to 7,400 years ago, Egypt 3,300 years ago and the western Asian steppes 5,500 years ago. Data on the origins of dairy farming in the eastern Asian steppes has been scant and the study by Jeong et al. (2018) addressed this problem.

These investigators analyzed fossil remains from the Khovsgol region, eastern steppes in Mongolia. The fossil remains were from the late Bronze Age dated 2,900 to 3,300 years ago. Genomic studies indicated that the Khovsgol remains contained about 11% ancient north Eurasian ancestry and between 4-7% western steppe herders ancestry and these studies indicated that there was a clear genetic separation between western steppe herder populations and late Bronze Age Mongolians. Jeong et al., (2018) also analyzed proteins found in the dental calculus of Khovsgol fossils and detected milk proteins specific for western domesticated ruminants. Hence ruminant dairy pastoralism was practiced in the eastern Asian steppes about 3,300 years ago. Despite the separation between western and eastern steppe populations, western dairy pastoralism was adopted by the eastern steppe population. Through a process of cultural exchange, western steppe populations introduced dairy pastoralism into eastern steppe populations. This scenario differs from what transpired in Europe where migration of outside populations including those of the western Asian steppes brought new technologies such as dairy farming i.e., demic diffusion (Orlando, 2018; Jeong et al., 2018).

An interesting sidelight of this study by Jeong et al. (2018) is that the Khovsgol fossils did not have the allele for lactase persistence consistent with the observation that lactase persistence is rare in modern Mongolians. In Europe and the Near East, dairy farming preceded the spread of the allele for lactase persistence by almost 5,000 years (Orlando, 2018; Jeong et al., 2018). These observations strongly suggest that dairy consumption in Europe and the Near East was not the only selective pressure that led to the spread of lactase persistence in these populations.

In the examples of cultural driven phenotypic changes described in the next sections, I have denoted the phenotype first followed by the underlying mechanism.

Lactase Persistence; Reciprocal Causation by Culture

Culture has the attribute of reciprocal causation; e.g., criterion 3 noted under definition of niche construction. For example, suppose a human population introduced an innovative cultural practice. That practice could modify the selection pressures acting on that population which in turn would elicit an evolutionary response through the action of natural selection in that population. In this example, the reciprocal causation attribute of culture acting through natural selection can lead to a phenotypic change in a population.

Examples of this mechanism include the genetic changes that occurred in humans following the introduction of different food sources (Laland et al., 2010). The classic example is that of milk consumption. Dairy farming with consumption of milk was introduced about 7,000 to 8,000 years ago. After introduction of this agricultural practice, there occurred a spread of the allele for lactase persistence within dairying populations. However, there are qualifications to this story which were discussed in the previous section.

Stone Tool Making; Cultural Inheritance

Although cultural inheritance and genetic inheritance have many parallels, there are some distinct differences (Creanza et al., 2017). Genetic transmission only occurs vertically between parents and offspring i.e., between generations. Cultural transmission, which occurs via social learning, can occur vertically from a parent, or nonparental adult, to a child i.e., between generations and also horizontally between individuals of the same generation. In genetics, gene mutations are the source of new traits while the origin of new cultural traits is more complex and poorly understood. Cultural novelty may arise through a trial and error learning process or through a novel combination of existing cultural traits. However, cultural and genetic inheritances should not be viewed as independent systems since the development and transmission of cultural traits are closely linked to the evolution of complex cognitive functions. A good example illustrating these links is the development of stone toolmaking during the Paleolithic period.

Stout (2011) reviewed the archaeological record of stone toolmaking during the Paleolithic period beginning about 2.6 million years ago. The earliest known stone tools are known as Oldowan tools, first found in Olduvai Gorge in Tanzania, and date to between 2.6 to 1.4 million years ago. These tools consisted of sharp stone flakes struck from a suitable core rock by direct percussion with another stone (the hammerstone). Tool production involved procuring the appropriate raw material i.e., core rock and hammerstone, followed by the actual flaking process. Flaking would have required a number of physical manipulations by the tool maker; grasping and rotating the core rock combined with a striking movement of the hammerstone.

About 1.6 million years ago, innovations in tool production took place. These more technologically advanced tools are known as Acheulean tools, first found in Saint-Acheul, France. Acheulean tools required more elaborate methods of flake production and these tools were intentionally shaped into large cutting tools, specifically large pointed hand axes and thick pointed picks. Late Acheulean large cutting tools (0.7 to 0.25 million years ago) were smaller, thinner, more regular and symmetrical. Production of these tools required a more elaborate shaping process involving a roughing-out and a finishing stage.

As Stout (2011) pointed out technological changes in tool making over the Paleolithic period were cumulative. The elaborate flake production and shaping methods used for making late Acheulean tools were built upon successive modifications made to previously established Oldowan and early Acheulean tool technologies. The foundation for the successful transmission of cumulative tool making behaviors across generations was the evolution of a hominin brain capable of complex cognitive functioning. In addition, sophisticated tool production required the acquisition of a set of pragmatic behavioral skills necessary for the actual physical process of tool making. A cognitively sophisticated hominin brain made possible the acquisition of such a set of skills through a combination of observation, experimentation and practice (Stout, 2017). Finally, as discussed in *Chapter 1*, culture was the primary driving force for the evolution of a large complex hominin brain.

In summary, a cultural practice such as tool making underscores the interdependence of cultural and genetic inheritance. Human culture selected out heritable variations in brain cognitive functions that promoted behaviors such as social learning, imitation and teaching that made possible the development of a progressively more elaborate culture. In the case of tool making, as the hominin brain became more sophisticated, social learning combined with cultural behaviors such as experimentation and practice allowed hominins to acquire the behavioral physical skills to make cumulative technological innovations in the construction of tools.

Put another way, one might have thought that transmission of a process such as toolmaking could be accounted for completely by cultural inheritance. However, the evolution of a progressively more elaborate tool making process required the co-evolution of a cognitively sophisticated brain and the co-evolution of the necessary physical skills to produce the tools. The message is that the processes of cultural inheritance and genetic inheritance generally cannot be separated.

Adaptation to a High Altitude; Hybridization

Hybridization is not generally viewed as a cultural practice. (See discussion in *Chapter 1* of hybridization as a speciation mechanism.) For example, hybridization events have been well documented in non-human species such as Darwin's finches (Lamichhaney et al., (2018). However, I believe past hybridization events in the human lineage should be viewed as cultural practices since these hybridization events resulted in distinct phenotypic outcomes.

Beall (2006) examined the adaptation of humans to a high altitude environment. Hypobaric hypoxia becomes progressively more severe with increasing altitude and populations that have colonized high altitude ecological niches have evolved various adaptations. Beall (2006) looked at three indigenous populations occupying the Andean, Tibetan and east African (Ethiopia) plateaus. Previous studies had indicated that the blood indices of humans of European ancestry living at altitudes of 1,600 metres (e.g., Rocky Mountains of the United States) and human populations in the Andes (altitude 4,000 metres) were characterized by an increased number of erythrocytes and an increased hemoglobin concentration. These adaptations allowed a given quantity of blood to carry more oxygen and would compensate for the low partial pressure of oxygen at that higher altitude.

However, studies in Tibetans living at 4,000 metres showed a different pattern of adaptations. A comparison of Andean and Tibetan samples collected from individuals living at 3,900 metres revealed that the Andean sample had a higher hemoglobin concentration than that of the Tibetan sample. A limited study of blood indices in Ethiopians residing at 3,530 metres showed a hemoglobin concentration comparable to that found at sea level. In Tibetans, only those living at altitudes of 5,000 metres showed an increase of hemoglobin concentration. Compared to Andean populations, Tibetans required a stronger hypobaric stimulus to increase hemoglobin concentration and their response was more blunted than that shown by Andean populations.

In essence, there appeared to be at least three different adaptation patterns (phenotypes) to a high altitude environment; a significant increase in hemoglobin concentration in Andean populations, a limited increase in hemoglobin concentration in Tibetan populations and apparently no change in hemoglobin concentration in Ethiopian populations.

The percentage of hemoglobin carrying oxygen (percent oxygen saturation) also differed between Andean and Tibetan populations (Beall, 2006). Populations at sea level had oxygen saturations of 97-98% while Andean populations at 4,000 metres had saturations of about 92% while Tibetan populations at 4,000 metres had saturations even lower at 89%. Ethiopians at 3,530 metres had a saturation of 95%. Beall (2006) noted that oxygen saturation had a significant heritability in the Tibetan population but not in the Andean population. An analysis of additional surveys indicated that this heritability in the Tibetan population reflected the effect of an autosomal dominant major gene and that presence of this major gene was associated with higher oxygen saturation of about 5-6%. The frequency of the high saturation allele ranged from 0.55 to 0.78 and this allele conferred a fitness advantage. Tibetan women homozygous or heterozygous for the high saturation allele and women homozygous for the low saturation allele all had the same number of live pregnancies. However, women homozygous or heterozygous for the high saturation allele had a significantly greater number of surviving children than women homozygous for the low saturation allele. This pattern would have led to spread of the high saturation allele throughout the population.

Recently, genomic studies have implicated the gene EPAS 1 (endothelial PAS domain protein 1) as the gene with the strongest signal of Tibetan specific selection for high altitude adaptation (Huerta-Sanchez et al., 2014). Human EPAS 1 encodes the oxygen sensitive subunit of the HIF (hypoxia-inducible –factor) -2 transcription factor and plays an important role in regulating erythropoiesis and level of hemoglobin (Hanaoka et al., 2012).

Huerta-Sanchez et al., (2014) sequenced the complete EPAS 1 gene in forty Tibetan and forty Han Chinese individuals. The EPAS 1 sequence variant they identified in the Tibetan group had a very low frequency in the

Han group and was absent from other modern human populations sampled. However, they found that the Tibetan allele was very similar to the allele carried by the archaic hominin species known as Denisovan. On the basis of these observations, Huerta-Sanchez et al., (2014) proposed that this Tibetan allele was introduced from Denisovan into humans prior to the divergence of Tibetan and Han populations about 54,000 years ago (Hu et al., 2017). This allele was then subject to natural selection when the separated Tibetan population colonized the high altitude plateau. This Tibetan specific allele functioned to regulate the physiological response to high altitude hypoxia, through the HIF signaling pathways, such as to maintain hemoglobin levels of Tibetan highlanders at near sea-level values (Hanaoka et al. 2012).

I would contend that this (gene) introgression from Denisovan to the human ancestor of Han and Tibetan populations should be viewed more broadly as evidence of ongoing cultural exchanges between Denisovan and humans. Clearly these cultural exchanges included mating. In fact there is considerable evidence for cultural exchanges between archaic hominins and between archaic hominins and humans. For example, recently a fossil fragment from Denisova cave in Russia was subjected to genomic sequencing. This analysis revealed that this fossil represented a first-generation Neanderthal-Denisovan offspring (Slon et al., 2018). As discussed in *Chapter 1,* genes introduced into humans through these cultural exchanges with archaic hominins have been associated with specific present day human phenotypes.

In this section, I have focused specifically on hybridization that occurred during cultural exchanges between Homo sapiens and other archaic hominins. However, these hybridization events took place in a much larger cultural context. As Homo sapiens migrated out of Africa and into the Levant and Europe, there occurred extensive cultural exchanges between Homo sapiens and Neanderthal. These two species had divergent cultures. Greenbaum et al., (2018) proposed that these extensive cultural exchanges were the primary driver responsible for the significant expansion of toolmaking and material culture that took place at the Middle

Paleolithic to Upper Paleolithic transition between 40, 000 to 50,000 years ago.

Migration and Variation in Skin Pigmentation; Phenotypic Plasticity

The ability of an organism to modify their phenotypes in response to environmental conditions is known as phenotypic plasticity (Perry et al., 2018). Recently, phenotypic plasticity has been incorporated into a theory of evolution, termed the plasticity-first hypothesis. In this construct, an environmentally induced phenotypic change (phenotypic plasticity) precedes and even facilitates evolutionary adaptation by natural selection (Levis and Pfennig, 2016).

An example of phenotypic plasticity was the phenomenon of industrial melanism in the peppered moth (Biston betularia). During the industrial revolution in Britain a previously unknown black form of the moth replaced the common pale type (van't Hof et al., 2011). The first black form of peppered moth was sighted in Manchester England in 1848. The emergence of this phenotypic change was driven by an interaction between avian predation and coal pollution. Black moths would be less visible to avian predators in an environment polluted by coal fumes. This initial plastic response selected for the insertion of a 22kb transposable element into the gene, Cortex which increased the transcriptional activity of this gene (van't Hof et al.; 2011, 2016). Within 20-30 moth generations this genetic variant had become widespread. This is an example of rapid evolution driven by phenotypic plasticity.

Is the geographical distribution of skin pigmentation in humans a manifestation of phenotypic plasticity? I believe so. Early archaic hominins after divergence from the common ancestor with chimpanzee and bonobo would have had hair covering most of their bodies (Jablonski and Chaplin, 2017). Rogers et al., (2004), based on genomic evidence, estimated that hominins first became hairless about 1.2 million years ago. Around that time, hominins were making extensive use of the African savannah and would have been actively hunting for prey. Active hunting practices in an open savannah environment (a new cultural practice) required an effective mechanism for thermoregulation. The mechanism that evolved was the loss of hair associated with the evolution of eccrine sweat glands covering most of the body. However, body hair had protected hominins from photodegradation of cutaneous and systemic folate by high ultraviolet radiation. Folate is an essential metabolite with important roles in DNA biosynthesis, embryonic development of the nervous system and maintenance of male fertility (Jablonski and Chaplin, 2017). It is believed that protection against folate photodegradation was the selective pressure that led to the evolution of dark protective eumelanin rich pigment in the skin. I suggest that the initial darkening of the skin was a plastic response to the loss of hair which protected the skin from the destructive effects of high ultraviolet radiation on folate. Following this initial plastic response, genetic accommodation occurred with adaptive selection of alleles providing additional protection of the skin from the sun i.e., plasticity preceded and facilitated adaptation by natural selection, with genes as followers.

Migration of Homo sapiens, starting about 60,000 years ago, into non-equatorial Africa, Eurasia and eventually the Americas exposed them to environments with less intense and more seasonally variable patterns of ultraviolet radiation (Jablonski and Chaplin, 2017). Ultraviolet radiation is important for catalyzing the production of vitamin D in the skin. In northern Eurasia, average ultraviolet radiation intensity is low and variable and dark skin pigmentation would have impaired cutaneous vitamin D production. The selective pressure in latitudes away from the equator would be for lesser skin pigmentation. Migration of humans into new environments away from the equator would have triggered a plastic response leading to lesser amounts of eumelanin in the skin. This plastic response was followed by selection of alleles adaptive for these new environments i.e., these derived alleles further modified the phenotype in the direction of the plastic response. In summary, the present day global geographical gradient of human skin pigmentation evolved through initial plastic responses followed by genetic changes and was driven by two competing selection pressures; protection against photodegradation of folate by ultraviolet radiation and production of cutaneous vitamin D by ultraviolet radiation.

The genetic underpinnings of present day geographical patterns of human skin pigmentation were recently analyzed by Martin et al., (2017). Since Africa is the home to the greatest range of pigmentation globally, Martin et al. (2017) chose as their study population the KhoeSan hunter-gatherers and pastoralists living in and near the Kalahari Desert in southern Africa. The term KhoeSan covered an array of indigenous populations in this area that were characterized by KhoeSan ancestry and the use of several specific languages. As part of this study, Martin et al., (2017) genotyped 465 KhoeSan individuals.

These investigators used narrow-band reflectometry to quantitate skin melanin content; a melanin index (M index) was derived from the percent red reflectance. A higher M index denoted darker skin pigmentation. They aggregated their KhoeSan skin pigmentation data with published data on thirty two globally diverse populations. Over this large database there was a strong inverse correlation between absolute latitude and skin pigmentation (M index). Populations further from the equator had a lower M index or lighter skin pigmentation. However, Martin et al., (2017) observed that the distribution or variance of skin pigmentation was greater in populations with darker skin than in populations with lighter skin. For example, the population in Ireland had a much lower M index than that of the near equatorial population of Ghana, but the distribution of M index values was much narrower in the Irish population compared to the Ghanaian population. The variance of M index across populations decreased with increasing distance from the equator. This observation probably reflects the genetic heterogeneity underlying skin pigmentation in different populations; lighter skin populations have less genetic heterogeneity than darker skin populations.

Using several different approaches, Martin et al. (2017) found that baseline (constitutive) skin pigmentation in the KhoeSan had a high degree of heritability. Based upon the KhoeSan genotype data, Martin et al., (2017) analyzed the genetic architecture underlying skin pigmentation in the KhoeSan. They looked at several gene sets. One was a gene set that consisted of 14 genes previously identified as associated with skin pigmentation e.g., SLC45A2, OCA2 and MC1R. A second set contained 50 genes with association to skin pigmentation based on more indirect methods and based on studies done in model organisms. A third gene set contained 50 genes associated with skin pigmentation in the KhoeSan based upon a GWAS (genome-wide association study) in the KhoeSan population. Martin et al., (2017) found that sets one and two accounted for a small fraction of the heritability of skin pigmentation in the KhoeSan. More of the heritability was explained by set three, but the rest of the genome (other than sets one, two or three) explained most of the heritability. Hence, skin pigmentation in KhoeSan was based upon an extensive polygenic architecture. In contrast, in European populations, predictive models based upon only nine alleles explained up to 16% of the heritability of skin pigmentation. In contrast, in the KhoeSan these same alleles had no predictive power.

In their study, Martin et al., (2017) noted that an allele of the gene SLC24A5 had a frequency of about 0.40 in the KhoeSan and was associated with lighter skin pigmentation. Recently, Lin et al., (2018) looked at the evolutionary history of this allele by sequencing the gene SLC24A5 to high coverage in two KhoeSan populations. This allele had a frequency of 0.33 in one population and 0.54 in the other. By comparison, In Northern Europeans this allele has a frequency of 1.00. The analysis of Lin et al., (2018) suggested the following sequence of events. This allele was introduced from migration of an Eastern African pastoralist population into southern Africa about 2,000 years ago. Subsequently, this allele was subjected to strong positive selection in the southern KhoeSan over the past 2,000 years. KhoeSan homozygous for this allele are 14% lighter in skin pigmentation than the population average. The adaptive advantage of this lighter skin pigmentation in the KhoeSan is not entirely clear although the southern tip of Africa receives relatively lower ultraviolet radiation intensity. This cultural exchange with gene flow from eastern pastoralists to southern KhoeSan was in a very broad sense comparable to the cultural exchange with gene flow from archaic Denisovan to humans.

In summary, the initial plastic change in skin pigmentation in equatorial African populations was followed by selection for multiple alleles with small effects. This polygenetic architecture was associated with wide intrapopulation distributions in melanin pigmentation and is consistent with a threshold model; the protective benefit of melanin needs to meet some minimum threshold with no penalty to darker pigmentation. Populations that migrated to regions far from the equator evolved lighter skin pigmentation. In these populations, the initial plastic response was followed by selection for fewer alleles with large effects. These populations had much narrower intrapopulation distributions in skin pigmentation. Populations at lesser distances from the equator showed genetic and variance characteristics between these two extremes.

A recent study in lizards provides an insight into potential mechanisms underlying plastic changes in coloration (Cori et al., 2018). Side-blotched lizards (Uta stansburiana) that inhabit the Pisgah Lava Flow in southern California exhibit a dark melanistic coloration that facilitates crypsis on dark volcanic rocks. This dark phenotype is distinct from nearby lizard populations that live on lighter colored soil and are more lightly colored. Both Pisgah and off-lava lizards become darker when housed for a year on lava. Lizards of both populations housed on lava become significantly lighter when switched to sand and conversely, lizards housed on sand become significantly darker when switched to lava. These observations demonstrate the plastic nature of the coloration phenotype in these lizards.

Because Pisgah lizards develop a darker coloration on lava then off-lava lizards housed on lava, the investigators questioned whether there was a genetic component to the coloration phenotype. Two candidate genes were identified; prolyl endopeptidase (PREP) and protein kinase cAMP-dependent type 1 regulatory subunit alpha (PRKAR1A). The protein products of these genes are involved in the synthesis of melanin. Comparison of single nucleotide polymorphisms (SNPs) between the two lizard populations identified derived alleles that were present in the Pisgah population but not the off-lava population. The investigators proposed that the derived alleles arose recently about 1,000 generations ago.

The data of Cori et al., (2018) suggested that the first lizards to colonize the Pisgah Lava flow developed a matching dark coloration to the lava background through ancestral plasticity in their skin coloration phenotype. Subsequently adaptive genetic changes occurred in the Pisgah population, particularly the emergence of derived alleles of genes PREP and PRKAR1A, which allowed these lizards to become even darker than that achieved through their initial plastic responses. Cori et al., (2018) proposed that ancestral plasticity in the coloration phenotype facilitated survival of lizards that colonized the lava environment and that the derived alleles of PREP and PRKAR1A originated after this colonization had occurred.

The data of Cori et al., (2018) can be used to describe a similar process in humans. Loss of hair in archaic hominins and migration of modern humans out of equatorial Africa created evolutionary pressures that elicited plastic skin coloration responses. This plasticity facilitated survival and was subsequently followed by adaptive genetic changes that further modified the phenotype in the direction of the plastic response.

Theory of Mind; Developmental Plasticity and Urbanization

Developmental plasticity, which was discussed in *Chapter 1,* is a variant of phenotypic plasticity. In this case, the environmental cue acts during a developmental stage. For example, as described in the Bucharest Early Intervention Project (Example 9, *Chapter 1*) lack of parental input at critical time points in the developmental process can induce lasting adverse phenotypic outcomes in offspring. Lack of parental input can be considered a poor cultural practice.

However, another example of culture and developmental plasticity involves the link between theory of mind and the origin of cities and a modern economy.

Humans possess a theory of mind which is a key cognitive attribute that guides our interactions with other humans. This cognitive attribute enables us to recognize that other humans have a set of beliefs, even false beliefs, that drive their behaviors (Tomasello, 2018). Agents behave not with respect to reality but with respect to their beliefs about reality. This cognitive attribute develops in early childhood and by age 4-5 years children begin to understand false beliefs (Tomasello, 2018).

Prior to the introduction of agriculture, humans lived as hunter-gatherers in small groups. The size of the group was such that an individual would have interacted directly with all other members of the group. These direct interactions would have been guided by an individual's understanding of the beliefs and thereby the behaviors of other individuals in the group. As pointed out by Boyer (2018) that type of direct interaction between an individual and all other members of the group was no longer possible when humans began to live in a large population such as a city and began to engage in economic activities such as trade and exchanges with individuals across long distances.

In a city, an individual interacts indirectly with most other humans living in that same city and the majority of these indirect interactions can be considered to be economic in nature. Since these interactions are indirect they can no longer be guided by one's theory of mind. Hence, living in a city and engaging in modern day economic activities required a change in our theory of mind such that we could trust the beliefs and thereby the intentions and behaviors of other humans that we did not interact with directly. Hence cultural practices such as living in a city and engaging in economic exchanges with others across large distances required the co-evolution of modifications to our theory of mind. In addition, living in cities required that we understand that core pieces of knowledge are possessed by everyone in the city; conventions, social norms and institutions apply to all individuals in the city and these parameters structure social interactions within the population.

One possibility is that the increasing urbanization of human populations and the introduction of trade and economic exchanges across distances elicited a plastic developmental change in our theory of mind, which made possible these cultural innovations. Following this plastic response, there would have occurred selection of alleles that further modified this cognitive attribute in that same direction. This possibility, however, is speculative on my part.

In this section, I have outlined examples in which human culture resulted in changes to human phenotypes. All of these phenotypic changes were accompanied by genomic changes except for the example involving development of a more expansive theory of mind. In this case, the occurrence of associated genomic changes is speculative on my part. Even though it may seem redundant, I think it is worthwhile to summarize these examples.

1. Through the introduction of new cultural practices, humans modify the selective pressures to which they are subjected. Natural selection acting on these altered evolutionary pressures can result in new phenotypic outcomes. Examples involving this mechanism include the introduction of dairy farming and other agricultural practices. These cultural practices made available new food sources and led to the selection of novel alleles such as the one for lactase persistence
2. The introduction of a novel cultural practice generally requires the co-evolution of new cognitive functions and/or new physical skills. Progressive sophistication of the stone tool making process required the co-evolution of enhanced cognitive functions and enhanced physical skills.
3. Archaic humans living and hunting in the open African savannah (a new cultural practice) evolved an effective thermoregulation mechanism which involved hair loss and development of a dense body distribution of sweat glands. Loss of hair exposed humans to photodegradation of folate by ultraviolet radiation. This selective pressure elicited an adaptive plastic response consisting of darkening skin pigmentation which protected humans from this destructive effect of ultraviolet radiation. This plastic response selected for multiple alleles which coded for darker skin coloration. When modern humans migrated out of equatorial Africa, a niche construction event, lighter skin pigmentation was

necessary to allow ultraviolet radiation to catalyze the production of cutaneous vitamin D. Migration to regions farther from the equator was associated with the evolution of progressively lighter skin coloration. The decrease in skin pigmentation was a plastic response which selected for additional alleles that coded for lighter skin coloration.

4. Appropriate parental care (described in Example 9, *Chapter 1*) at specific stages of development is critical to offspring phenotypic outcomes. As described in the example of the Bucharest Early Intervention Project, a cultural practice such as lack of parental care at critical developmental stages can have adverse effects on offspring phenotypic outcomes since development is a plastic process. These adverse effects can last for the life time of the offspring. Studies using the rat mother-pup model, also discussed in Example 9, indicate that maternal care can be associated with epigenetic changes in offspring.

A second example linking culture and developmental plasticity is the association between theory of mind and origin of cities and a modern economy. Living in cities and engaging in modern economic activities meant that most interactions between an individual and others would be indirect and hence could not be guided by one's theory of mind. Initially a plastic response in theory of mind enabled an individual to trust the beliefs and thereby the intentions and behaviors of others with whom that individual did not directly interact. I have speculated that subsequent selection of alleles further modified theory of mind in that same direction.

5. In the remote past, cultural exchanges between humans and other hominin groups resulted in gene introgression with lasting phenotypic changes. One gene acquired from Denivosan has been pivotal in enabling Tibetans to successfully live at high altitudes.

In these examples, cultural and genetic inheritances are tightly interconnected. In the next section, I describe examples of cultural driven phenotypic changes without associated genomic changes. These phenotypic changes have occurred very recently and their mechanism of inheritance may simply be through cultural inheritance without any subsequent selection for novel alleles. However, it could be that the timelines are too short for genetic changes to have occurred.

CULTURE DRIVEN PHENOTYPIC CHANGES WITH NO OBVIOUS ASSOCIATED GENOMIC CHANGES

In this section, I will describe examples in which cultural practices have resulted in phenotypic changes without any obvious accompanying genomic changes. These examples illustrate the effects of two culturally driven mechanisms not described in the previous section. One mechanism, involves the cultural practice of defining ranges of normal for human traits, both physiological and behavioral. In essence, this practice determines for that cultural group what constitutes an adaptive or non-adaptive trait. Since culturally defined norms will differ between cultural groups so will what is considered normal (adaptive) and abnormal (non-adaptive). A behavior that is considered normal (adaptive) in one cultural group may be considered abnormal (non-adaptive) in another cultural group.

A second mechanism involves the action of a cultural practice to modify physiological traits, either inadvertently or purposely, and through this modification change phenotypes.

Both mechanisms are evident in the examples discussed in this section.

Attention Deficit Hyperactivity Disorder (ADHD)

Much of present day human culture is highly technological with particular aspects being the domains of communication including social media and transfer of information. However, as reviewed by Meyer (2018) the modern digital information era actually began around the year 1440 with the construction of moveable-type printing presses by Guttenberg and others. The IBM 704 mainframe was introduced in 1954 and the internet had its beginnings in the late 1960s and early 1970s. In the early 1990s the World Wide Web was introduced to the public by scientists at CERN, the European Organization of Nuclear Research. Since then there has been an explosion of technological advances including; personal computers, smart phones, email, search engines and social media platforms to name a few. However, concerns have been raised as to the effects of this new informational environment, fueled by these myriad of digital devices, on child development (Meyer, 2018).

ADHD is considered to be a continuum of a set of ADHD-related behaviors; attention problems, hyperactivity and impulsivity. The prevalence of this disorder has increased by as much as 30% over the past 20 years (Christakis et al., 2018). Beyens et al., (2018) reviewed published data on the relationship between media use in children and adolescents and ADHD-related behaviors. Media use included television viewing and video game playing, both violent and nonviolent. Recently, a model has been proposed which defined potential links between media use and ADHD-behaviors. This model advanced three propositions. a) Media effects are indirect and are mediated by their influence on cognitive, emotional and excitative response states in an individual. b) Individuals vary in their susceptibility to media effects. c) The effects of media use in susceptible individuals lead to subsequent media use in those individuals i.e., media use is self-reinforcing. Beyens et al., (2018) used this model as a metric for evaluating published studies. They found that most of the published studies were correlational in nature and did not address potential mechanisms linking media use and ADHD-related behaviors as proposed in the model. Beyens et al. (2018) concluded that currently published studies did support a relationship between media use in children and adolescents and ADHD-related behaviors, that the statistical significance of this relationship was small, but that none of these studies looked at underlying mechanisms.

Christakis et al., (2018) looked at links between media use and ADHD-related behaviors from the perspective of neurodevelopment. Christakis et al., (2018) noted that children today begin watching television at a very young age, about 4 months. Young children today are also exposed to smart phones, tablets and computers. The question raised by these investigators is what effects might the use of digital media in early life have on neurodevelopment?

Cortical development involves a number of processes. Formation of neurons and their migration occur prenatally. Arborization (circuit formation) and myelination begin prenatally but continue through the first 20 years after birth. Full development and functionality of the human brain takes more than 20 years, but the first few years of life are considered the most crucial (Christakis et al., 2018). Environmental cues can have a significant influence on this neurodevelopmental process (developmental plasticity). For example animals reared in a complex and enriched environment show much different neurodevelopmental outcomes than animals reared in an impoverished environment (Christakis et al., 2018). These observations indicate that environmental stimulation can have a beneficial effect on brain development. But can the brain be overstimulated i.e., can too much sensory stimulation lead to adverse neurodevelopmental outcomes?

Christakis et al., (2018) developed a mouse model to look at the behavioral effects of excessive sensory stimulation (ESS). The experimental setup was as follows. Mice received an ESS experience for 6 hours per day for 42 days. ESS was delivered by speakers mounted above standard mouse cages and colored lights positioned on all four walls. Audio was piped in at 70 dB, levels typical of television watching but less than the 100-115dB that causes acoustic stress in mice. Colors and intensities were changed in concordance with the audio to simulate television watching. On postnatal day 10, mice were divided into two groups; a control group and an experimental group exposed to ESS as outlined. Mice from both groups remained with their mother until weaning (postnatal day 21) and then were housed in groups of up to five mice per cage. Ten days after cessation of ESS, both groups of mice were subjected to a battery of behavioral tests.

Anxiety, learning and memory were decreased, whereas risk taking and motor activity were enhanced in ESS mice compared to controls. In other words, ESS mice were hyperkinetic and less risk averse compared to control mice. It is important to remember that the ESS was delivered without social isolation. ESS and control mice had comparable parental care and were housed in cages with similar numbers of mice. These behavioral changes were associated with alterations in glutamatergic transmission in the nucleus accumbens and amygdala.

These experimental observations are consistent with previous work done by these investigators in children. Increased television viewing before the age of three, was associated with increased risk of attentional problems at school age. In addition, faster pacing of shows gave stronger associations with subsequent attentional problems.

In summary, observations in children and experimental observations in very young mice indicate that excessive sensory stimulation, as would be provided by current patterns of television viewing, can alter neurodevelopment in the direction of ADHD-like behaviors. In essence, excessive media exposure, a present day cultural practice, induces a neurodevelopmental plastic response leading to an altered behavioral phenotype.

The potential impact of excessive sensory stimulation on neurobiological functions can be appreciated by examining how the brain processes sensory stimuli. Recently, the code that the brain uses to recognize faces from a multitude of small differences in shapes, distances between features, skin tones and textures has been elucidated (Abbott, 2018). The brain areas involved in facial recognition include the visual cortex, where information first arrives from the retina, and the inferior temporal (IT) cortex. Studies in non-human primates have identified in the IT cortex patches of neurons which respond to facial features. Neurons located in patches at the top of the IT cortex, responded to shape parameters such as the distance between eyes, width of a mouth or shape of a hairline. Neurons in patches deeper in the IT cortex responded to appearances such as skin tone and texture. These differential bits of facial information elicit responses from specific patch neurons as well as eliciting differences in firing frequency. For example, a neuron responding to the distance between eyes would have a firing rate related to whether the eyes are close-set or farther apart. This system, by using all of these dimensions of "faceness", generates an internal image of a particular face. One could speculate that this code-type mechanism for processing visual information about faces, could represent a model as to how other sensory stimuli (auditory, tactile, taste) are processed by the brain. In sum total, the brain processes multiple sensory stimuli to generate an internal version of external reality. In addition, Abbott (2018) described a current model, referred to as predictive processing, whereby the brain operates by predicting how its immediate surroundings will change millisecond by millisecond and compares this prediction with the information it receives through various senses. The brain uses any mismatches to update its version of external reality.

Given this model of how the brain generates an updated internal version of external reality, one can conceive of different scenarios in which excessive sensory stimulation by distorting this sensory processing system could lead to adverse behavioral phenotypes. For example, exposure of a young child whose brain is still maturing to excessive sensory stimulation could result in faulty development of this sensory processing system. Exposure of an adult to excessive sensory stimulation could significantly perturb inputs into this sensory mechanism and thereby lead to distortions in the internal image of external reality generated by the brain.

A cautionary note is in order. In this section I have looked specifically at the relationship between media use and ADHD like behaviors. In other studies, researchers looked at the use of digital technology in adolescents and found very little effect on overall well-being (Editorial, 2019). However, I suspect that overall well-being is too general an outcome measure and that the effects of digital technology target more specific cognitive/behavioral functions.

Schizophrenia

Schizophrenia was first recognized as a separate diagnostic entity about one hundred years ago although the initial diagnostic term was dementia praecox (Insel, 2010). In the early twentieth century the term schizophrenia was proposed and this disease was considered to be a fundamental disorder of thought and feeling. Insel (2010) has proposed that schizophrenia be considered a neurodevelopmental disorder and as such could be divided into stages. This neurodevelopmental model posited that the trajectory of this disorder begins in the prenatal or perinatal period. In adolescence a prodromal second stage has been described based upon the occurrence of bizarre thoughts, social isolation and impaired functioning. Schizophrenic psychosis, stage three, usually emerged between ages 18 to 25 years and was followed by a stage of chronic disability, stage four. Chronic schizophrenia is associated with a number of medical complications including metabolic syndrome in 40% and a reduced life expectancy. Insel (2010) suggested that schizophrenia may actually be many different disorders with different outcomes.

One of the primary neurodevelopmental attributes impaired in schizophrenia is theory of mind. Brune (2005) reviewed the published literature on the topic of theory of mind research in schizophrenia. There is abundant evidence that patients with schizophrenia have impaired theory of mind but it is not clear if an impaired theory of mind is the primary developmental abnormality in schizophrenia or at what stage this impairment emerges.

Impaired theory of mind has been identified as a feature of other neuropsychiatric disorders such as autism spectrum disorder and bipolar disorder (Brewer et al., 2017; Mitchell and Young, 2016). These observations lead to a logical question. Why is theory of mind such an important neurodevelopmental attribute? To address this question, we need to examine theory of mind in more detail.

Theory of Mind

There are a number of definitions of theory of mind but one definition is the ability to attribute mental states –beliefs, intents, desires, knowledge and so forth –to oneself and others and to understand that others have beliefs, desires and intentions that are different from one's own (Westby, 2014). According to Tomasello (2018), the core feature of the theory of mind is beliefs; individuals behave not with respect to reality but with respect to their beliefs about reality. Beliefs are mental representations that their possessor takes to correspond to an objective reality. However, an individual could hold a false belief and thus the individual could be acting rationally from his/her subjective perspective but irrationally from an objective reality perspective (Tomasello, 2018). Children begin to recognize false beliefs around ages 4- 5 years.

Theory of mind has a deep evolutionary history since our closet non-human primates, the great apes, have an ancestral-type theory of mind (Tomasello, 2018). Within species of great apes, theory of mind allowed an individual to imagine and track the mental states and intentions of others in the context of social competition. This cognitive attribute allowed an individual to make predictions about a competitor's intentions and behaviors and making such predictions did not require an individual to determine whether a competitor's mental state was based upon a false belief. This ancestral theory of mind allowed social animals to compete successfully with conspecifics for food, resources and mates. In contrast, the human lineage evolved highly cooperative social interactions which have enabled our species to live in large cities and to engage in global economic activity. Tomasello (2018) proposed that the evolution of our cooperative behavior was based upon shared intentionality i.e., sharing of activities and goals with others and required a more elaborate theory of mind. In the context of shared intentionality, an individual would want his/her partner to be able to read his/her mind. However, to guard against the possibility that a partner might take advantage of such a cooperative situation by lying or deceiving it is important that an individual be able to recognize false beliefs in a partner.

The traditional view has been that theory of mind in humans was a unitary construct dependent upon cognitive abilities. The construct discussed in the previous section focused on the ability of an individual to cognitively assess the intentions and beliefs of others. However more recent studies in humans have indicated that theory of mind is actually a multidimensional construct involving not only beliefs and intentions but also emotional states (Westby, 2014) i.e., an individual can decipher not only the intentions and beliefs of others but also their emotional states. Theory of mind has been further differentiated into intrapersonal when one is thinking about one's own beliefs and emotions and interpersonal when one is thinking about the beliefs and emotions of others.

Dvash and Shamay-Tsoory (2014) have examined the neurobiological evidence supporting what has been termed affective theory of mind. They further classified affective theory of mind into two categories; cognitive affective theory of mind which focuses on an individual's cognitive assessment of the emotional states of others and affective empathy which is the, largely unconscious, ability of an individual to respond to the emotional states of others.

In summary, cognitive theory of mind involves interpreting thoughts, intentions and beliefs of others while affective theory of mind involves thinking about feelings and emotional states of others. Affective empathy can be regarded as an emotional reaction of an individual to another individual when perceiving that the other individual is experiencing or is about to experience an emotion. In the human empathy is to be viewed as a component of theory of mind.

Related to the construct of intrapersonal theory of mind is autobiographical memory (Westby, 2014). Autobiographical memory is defined as explicit memory for specific points in the past recalled from the perspective of the self in relation to others i.e., it involves a sense of self through time and is the foundation for intrapersonal theory of mind. One of the determinants of the richness of autobiographical memory is how mothers reminisce with their young children. Mothers who are more elaborative in their reminiscences have children with a more detailed representation of both past events and the links between previous internal mental states and current internal mental states and behaviors. A better developed intrapersonal theory of mind helps an individual better assess the mental states of others (Westby, 2014).

There is also an important role of language in a child's development of theory of mind (de Villiers and de Villiers, 2014). A child's interactions with other individuals are greatly enriched by the acquisition of language skills. Language skills give children a greater understanding of the perspective others bring to the conversation and more conversation in rich social contexts allows meanings for words defining mental states to emerge. Language is a tool that allows a child to compare and contrast his/her own beliefs and knowledge with those of others. Children with language impairment or who are deaf show delayed attainment of theory of mind as well as reduced quality of autobiographical memory (Westby, 2014).

In this discussion of theory of mind the setting has been direct interactions between individuals. Such a direct interaction allows an individual to use verbal language and body language as cues to aid in deciphering the beliefs, knowledge and intentions of others with who that individual is directly interacting. But in our modern society most interactions between individuals are not face-to-face but indirect. These interactions are generally of an economic nature.

An example would be as follows. You are planning to fly from your present location to another destination. During this whole process the number of individuals you directly interact with is very limited. You most likely purchase the airline ticket online, but you would interact directly with several individuals when you check in to the airline desk and deposit baggage. However, you do not directly interact with the individuals who put your baggage on the airplane, the pilots who fly the airplane, the myriad of individuals who built, maintain and test the airplane. The point is that in our present day urban society we cannot apply theory of mind to assess the beliefs, intentions and emotional states of the great majority of individuals with whom we interact since these interactions are all indirect. How then do we decide whether we can trust these individuals? After all, if the airplane you take has not been properly built or serviced, there could be a fatal accident. We have had to develop what I will call an extended theory of mind to enable us to trust the thousands of individuals we interact with only indirectly, usually for economic transactions. Such an extended theory of mind is necessary to allow human populations living in cities, states and countries to function in a manner that is both orderly and mutually advantageous for the citizenry. This extended theory of mind enables an individual living in an urban setting to willing accept that the beliefs, intentions and emotional states of other individuals that he/she interacts with only indirectly are most likely congruent with his/her own beliefs, intentions and emotional states.

Stanzione and Schick (2014) looked at environmental cues that influence the development of theory of mind. Similar to the views of Dvash and Shamay-Tsoory (2014) these investigators pointed out that theory of mind is an expansive developmental process involving a range of steps beginning early in life with the more complex aspects, such as understanding of false beliefs, emerging around age 4-5 years.

Stanzione and Schick (2014) noted that using understanding of false beliefs as a measuring tool, theory of mind appeared to be a universal attribute across different cultures.

To look at the influence of language on theory of mind, they compared two groups of children; children who are deaf or hard-of hearing (DHH) whose parents are also DHH and children who are DHH but have hearing parents. DHH children who have DHH parents typically grow up in a language rich environment since children and parents generally share a common sign language. In contrast DHH children who have hearing parents generally develop in language environments that have limited access to spoken language and have parents who are typically not fluent in sign language. DHH children with DHH parents performed equally well as hearing children in their false-belief performance whereas DHH children with hearing parents were delayed in their acquisition of false belief understanding with only a 50% group success rate at 7 years of age. Additional studies indicated that DHH children with hearing parents continued to develop theory of mind into adulthood, although evidence of delays persisted. These observations suggest that children with DHH and hearing parents have fewer experiences with conversational interactions that involve mental state and emotional terms and thereby have impaired development of theory of mind.

Stanzione and Schick (2014) reported a relationship between socioeconomic status and children's theory of mind. Children growing up in low socioeconomic families performed worse on theory of mind tasks than children who grew up in working class families or families of professional status. There are a number of factors underlying this relationship and one such factor would be the richer conversational milieu that would be found in families of higher socioeconomic status.

Colvert et al. (2008) measured theory of mind in Romanian orphans who had been subjected to extreme social isolation in early life (see Example 9, in *Chapter 1*). These children showed deficits in theory of mind tasks, with degree of impairment being greater in children who had experienced more than six months of institutional deprivation.

In summary, theory of mind is a neurodevelopmental attribute that enables an individual to recognize that he/she and others have beliefs, intentions and emotional states that may be similar or different. It also enables an individual to recognize that others act on the basis of their beliefs even if those beliefs are false i.e., counter to objective reality. Theory of mind develops in stages in young children and by age 4-5 years, a child has learned to recognize that others can have false beliefs and can act on the basis of those false beliefs. The developmental stages for theory of mind are intimately linked to acquisition of language skills and individuals who grow up in an environment of sparse conversational interactions with parents have impaired theory of mind.

Our closest primate relatives have an ancestral theory of mind which allows them to track the knowledge states and intentions of conspecifics. This ancestral theory of mind allows non-human primates to make predictions about a conspecific's behavior, an ability that is beneficial in the context of competition for food, resources and mates. However, non-human primates lack an understanding of false beliefs. We have evolved a much more multidimensional theory of mind which allows us to track the beliefs (both true and false), intentions and emotional states of other humans. Language skills and the richness of parental conversations focusing on mental states and emotions, including autobiographical memory, are important factors in children's development of theory of mind. The evolution of our theory of mind was based upon shared intentionality i.e., humans often openly share goals, beliefs and emotional states with others thus promoting cooperativity. Theory of mind is a critical neurodevelopmental attribute that forms the foundation for our social interactions and culture. As discussed in *Chapter 1*, culture has driven the evolution of a cognitively sophisticated brain which in turn has enabled us to develop a progressively more elaborate cumulative culture. I would contend that culture has specifically driven the evolution of theory of mind as a critical cognitive attribute that made possible the everyday social interactions that form the basis of culture.

The evolution of theory of mind is foundational to the creation of culture and *schizophrenia* can be considered the *biological cost of culture*. Failure of an individual to develop a functionally normal theory of mind results in that individual being unable to engage in appropriate social interactions with other humans which manifests as a neuropsychiatric disorder such as schizophrenia. However, I refer to schizophrenic-like behavior as a biological cost because this behavioral variant is only apparent within the context of culture.

There is evidence in support of this proposal. Krabbendam and van Os (2005) reviewed the results of ten studies that compared the rate of schizophrenia in urban compared to rural areas. Cities have a higher density of people and a richer level of social interactions than rural areas. Most of these studies adjusted for various socioeconomic variables that could have influenced the results. The authors performed a meta-analysis of these studies and found that the rate of schizophrenia in urban areas was around double that in rural areas. They noted that the urban versus rural difference was consistent across countries and cultures and many studies demonstrated a dose –response relationship between extent of urbanization and rate of schizophrenia. Krabbendam and van Os (2005) concluded that this was a true association between urbanicity and rate of schizophrenia and not due to factors such as more people with a genetic liability for schizophrenia moving into cities. The authors suggested that there was a gene –environment interaction between an urban environment and an underlying genetic predisposition although they could not identify what was specific about an urban exposure.

I do not propose that culture "causes" schizophrenia. A number of foundational neurodevelopmental processes co-evolved with and made possible the emergence of a highly sophisticated human cumulative culture as discussed in *Chapters 1 and 3*. Social learning enhanced through the use of symbolic language and teaching allowed culture to be transmitted across generations with high fidelity. A multidimensional theory of mind which enabled an individual to tap into the beliefs and emotional states of others, and to empathize with others, allowed humans to engage in the highly social and cooperative interactions that made culture possible. My contention is that since culture has become more and more socially interactive through urbanization and globalization, individuals who have impaired theory of mind for whatever reason cannot function within our prevailing culture i.e., they cannot engage in normal social interactions with others and manifest behaviors that we label as schizophrenia or bi-polar disorder or autism spectrum disorder. Schizophrenia and other neuropsychiatric disorders with impaired theory of mind can only exist within the context of culture.

In essence, the cultural practice of setting boundaries defining norms for human traits, both physiological and behavioral, establishes what is normal (adaptive) and what is abnormal (non-adaptive). In other words, a cultural group develops a consensus as to what constitutes normal and abnormal behaviors. These norms will differ from culture to culture and as a result what constitutes normal and abnormal behaviors will differ from culture to culture.

Within this framework, one could make several predictions. Non-human primates, who have a simpler theory of mind that does not tap into false beliefs or emotional states of conspecifics, would not manifest schizophrenic-type behaviors. There is not data available to test this prediction. City dwellers exposed to a higher "dose" of culture than rural dwellers would have a higher rate of schizophrenia than rural dwellers. Studies supporting this prediction were discussed in a previous paragraph. In the next section, we will look at the role of genomic studies in schizophrenia.

Genomic Studies

There have been a number of genome -wide association studies (GWAS) in schizophrenia looking for genetic variants linked to this disorder and as for most complex traits, the risk profile is highly polygenic

Visscher et al., 2017). Recently a PyschENCODE Consortium was formed to characterize the full spectrum of genomic elements within the human brain that play a role in development and neuropsychiatric disorders such as schizophrenia (The PsychCONSORTIUM, 2018).

Rajarajan et al., (2018) looked at the three dimensional structure of the genome. Chromatin is not organized in a linear fashion but in a hierarchical arrangement that can bring widely separated DNA regions into close approximation. As their model system, these investigators generated neural progenitor cells (NPCs) from induced human pluripotent stem cells and monitored the differentiation of these NPCs into neurons or astrocyte-like glial cells. Using this in vitro model of brain development, they mapped cell-type specific chromatin conformations associated with schizophrenic risk loci. For neuron specific interactions, Rajarajan et al., (2018) identified 158 genes within risk loci but another 227 genes located outside risk loci but connected via intrachromatin contacts with risk loci. Similarly, for NPC specific and glial specific interactions they identified genes that were within risk loci and genes that were outside risk loci but connected to risk loci through chromatin conformational arrangements. On the basis of these findings, the investigators were able to greatly expand the number of risk genes to include not only genes directly in risk loci but also genes connected to the risk loci through interactions created by the three dimensional structure of the genome. Hence, by looking at the three dimensional genome, the investigators were able to expand the number schizophrenic risk genes by 50-150% depending on the cell type i.e., NPC, neuron or glial cell.

Gandal et al., (2018) looked at gene expression using RNA sequencing in post mortem brain samples, frontal and temporal cortex, from individuals with schizophrenia, autism spectrum disorder and bipolar disorder as well as controls. Gene expression was measured at several levels; gene level, transcript isoform expression, local splicing and coexpression networks for both protein coding and non-protein coding genes. Expression changes at the level of transcript isoforms, as opposed to the gene level, showed the largest effect sizes and the greatest disease specificity. For example, differential changes in the expression of distinct transcript isoforms of more than 50 genes were noted in schizophrenia. In schizophrenic brains, 693 noncoding RNAs were differentially expressed. The investigators identified gene and transcript isoform coexpression networks and of 90 coexpression networks, 36 showed patterns of dysregulation specific to one of the three psychiatric disorders.

These two studies highlight the widespread genomic changes that are found in the brains of individuals labeled with a neuropsychiatric disorder such as schizophrenia. Taking account of the three dimensional organization of chromatin, Rajarajan et al. (2018) were able to identify many more risk genes for schizophrenia than had previously been identified. In the brains of those labeled with neuropsychiatric disorders, changes in gene expression at the transcript isoform level had a much bigger effect and were more disease specific than those at the level of the gene. However, these genomic changes cannot be used to define specific neuropsychiatric disorders since they cannot be directly translated into specific phenotypes. Defining a specific disorder can only be done at the phenotypic level. But, these genomic changes can give us clues as to how specific neural molecular processes vary between individuals we classify as normal and individuals we label as schizophrenic.

In summary, within a population there will be variations in theory of mind between individuals based upon genomic variants and differential exposures to environmental cues e.g., parental influences, during neural development. These variations in theory of mind will lead to variations in the capacity of individuals to engage in highly cooperative social interactions with others. If an individual's social behaviors fall outside agreed upon culturally defined population norms then that individual will be labeled as suffering from a neuropsychiatric disorder such as schizophrenia. My contention is that the more highly complex and urbanized the culture is, the more restricted in range will be the agreed upon norms for social behaviors. This more restricted range will result in a higher rate for culturally defined neuropsychiatric disorders.

Metabolic Diseases: Obesity, Type 2 Diabetes

Obesity has been discussed in medical writings dating back to the time of Hippocrates (Bray, 1990). These writings included advice about dietary restrictions and exercise as treatments but these treatments were framed within the concept that obesity represented moral weakness on the part of the obese individual. However, over the past 50 years obesity and type 2 diabetes have reached epidemic proportions. In 2011-2012 more than one third of the population of the United States was obese (Bhupathiraju and Hu, 2016). In the case of type 2 diabetes the primary problem is insulin resistance. In a lengthy review, Petersen and Shulman (2018) discussed the mechanisms of insulin action and insulin resistance. Quoting from their paper; "The fundamental element linking all putative mediators of insulin resistance is a relationship to nutrient oversupply."

My purpose is not to review the biology of obesity and type 2 diabetes. The literature on these topics is very extensive. My focus instead is on the role culture has played in the current obesity-diabetes epidemic. Since nutrient oversupply is a foundational element for both obesity and diabetes, I will focus on how culture has influenced eating behaviors and obesity.

Evolutionary Background

Sellayah et al., (2014) examined the evolutionary roots of human obesity. Prior to plant and animal domestication and the introduction of agriculture, hunter gatherers were subject to fluctuations in food supply. According to the "thrifty gene hypothesis", the action of natural selection resulted in the emergence of genes that favored energy storage i.e., thrifty genes. These alleles enabled humans to store food as fat during periods of food abundance in order to provide for periods of food shortage. During a period of food abundance, as exists now, thrifty genes would result in population obesity. According to Sellayah et al., (2014), the "thrifty gene hypothesis" has a number of shortcomings and these investigators have proposed a different evolutionary origin for obesity.

They postulated that selection factors related to climate underlie the obesity phenotype. As humans migrated out of Africa about 60,000 to

70,000 years ago, they would have encountered different climatic conditions. Those exposed to colder environments evolved enhanced cold adaptation mechanisms. These mechanisms involved brown adipose tissue (BAT) which is a source of heat production. In response to cold, BAT breaks down stored triglycerides into free fatty acids (FFAs) and glycerol. FFAs enter BAT mitochondria and activate uncoupling protein 1, which uncouples ATP synthesis from oxidative phosphorylation. This process produces heat via an energy wastage mechanism. Genes that augment BAT function would be advantageous in cold climates. Sellayah et al., (2014) proposed that migration to northern latitudes would have resulted in selection of genes for cold adaptation i.e., increased metabolic rate and enhanced BAT function. Ancestral humans who remained in hot (tropical) climates evolved mechanisms for heat adaptation such as a reduced metabolic rate. In essence, climatic selection pressures strongly influenced gene selection for either efficient cold or warm adaptation. According to this proposal, cold versus warm heat adaptation, with their differing metabolic profiles, was the evolutionary basis for why obesity has had a differential prevalence across cultures within the pat 50-75 years. Human populations that are cold adapted are at a reduced risk to develop obesity compared to populations that are heat adapted.

West-Eberhard (2019) recently outlined a different perspective on the evolutionary origins of obesity. This perspective is based upon two observations. First, visceral (omental and mesenteric) fat and not subcutaneous fat is the adipose tissue associated with chronic inflammatory disorders such as obesity, and type 2 diabetes and secondly poor nutrition during fetal development is associated in adulthood with these same chronic inflammatory diseases particularly in those individuals whose food input was increased later. Visceral adipose tissue (VAT) is metabolically more active than subcutaneous adipose tissue (SAT) and also has important immune functions. VAT acts as a defense mechanism against intraperitoneal pathogens and foreign matter. Infants and children who were exposed to poor fetal nutrition (fetal nutritional stress) are at increased risk for infections whereas infants and children who were well nourished during fetal development are better able to resist infection.

Based upon this observation, West-Eberhard (2019) proposed that individuals subjected to poor fetal nutrition would favor investment in VAT whereas individuals well-nourished during fetal development would favor investment in SAT. When individuals subjected to fetal nutritional stress are later given increased nutrition, they have a high risk of developing obesity and type 2 diabetes, due to their investment in VAT. In this scenario, VAT obesity leads to an altered immune response which triggers a chronic inflammatory state and increasing insulin resistance.

West-Eberhard (2019) put these observations into an evolutionary framework. Perhaps the first investment in VAT came with animal domestication and creation of large settlements. Under these conditions, humans were exposed to infectious microbes transmitted from domesticated animals and between humans living closely together. This transmission was facilitated by the unsanitary conditions that existed in early settlements. With the emergence of civilizations, there developed societal stratification with increased socioeconomic and health inequalities. VAT investment would have been favored in low resource individuals, those at the lowest rung of the socioeconomic ladder, who would have been exposed to fetal nutritional stress. These individuals would have been at increased risk to develop VAT obesity and related chronic inflammatory conditions. In essence, the VAT hypothesis links poor nutrition during fetal development to the emergence, over the past 10,000 years, of stratified societies characterized by increasing resource inequalities. Poor fetal nutrition within the population occupying the lower socioeconomic levels led to VAT investment in this population. For the reasons discussed, VAT investment put this population at a high risk to develop VAT obesity, type 2 diabetes and cardiovascular disease.

In summary, there are at least three hypotheses as to the evolutionary origins of the present epidemic of obesity and type 2 diabetes. The "thrifty gene" and cold/heat adaptation hypotheses describe genetic selection processes that had their origins at least 70,000 years ago. The VAT investment hypothesis traces the genetic origins of obesity and type 2 diabetes to the period of the Neolithic revolution, about 10,000 years ago, when domestication of animals occurred and agriculture was introduced.

All three hypotheses provide a mechanism, albeit different ones, by which excess food intake can lead to obesity. In the "thrifty gene" hypothesis, populations enriched for thrifty genes will preferentially store excess food as fat. In the cold/heat adaptation hypothesis, populations with a greater degree of heat adaptation and thereby a lower metabolic rate will preferentially store excess food as fat. In the VAT investment hypothesis, populations exposed to fetal nutritional stress will invest in enhanced VAT functions. These populations will preferentially store excess food in VAT with the development of visceral obesity.

At this juncture it is useful to return to the Tsimane population living in Bolivia as a yardstick for assessing the prevalence of obesity and chronic inflammatory diseases in humans about 10,000 years ago. As discussed in *Chapter 1*, the Tsimane are an indigenous population of forager-horticulturalists living in Bolivia. Kaplan et al., (2017) studied 705 individuals ranging in age between 40-94 years during the years 2014-2015. There was an equal split between males and females and since no gender bias was found the data from males and females were combined. At the population level, the prevalence of obesity, coronary artery disease and hypertension were extremely low. Coronary artery disease is currently considered to be a chronic inflammatory disease. Mean body mass index (BMI) in those 40-44 years old was 23.7 kg/m^2 and 24.1 kg/m^2 in those 75 years and older. Only three percent of those aged 40-44 years had a BMI greater than 30 kg/m2 and in those 75 years and older only two percent had a BMI greater than 30 kg/m^2. Mean body fat (%) was 21.8 in those aged 40-44 years and 21.7 (%) in those aged 75 years and older. Kaplan et al. (2017) also measured inflammatory markers. Mean high sensitivity C-reactive protein (CRP) was 3.2 mg/L in those aged 40-44 years and 4.0 mg/L in those aged 75 years and older. A value of 3.0 mg/L is the upper cutoff for CRP and 43% of those aged 40-44 years and 45% of those aged 75 years and older had a value above 3.0 mg/L. For erythrocyte sedimentation rate (ESR), 30% of those aged 40-44 years and 41% of those aged 75 years and older had a value above the upper cutoff of 22 mm/h. These measures of ESR and CRP indicated that Tsimane had a high inflammatory burden, presumably infectious in origin. Over two thirds of adults suffer from intestinal helminths at any given time. In addition, the levels of ESR and inflammatory markers interleukin 5 and interleukin 10 were inversely proportional to coronary artery calcification scores i.e., higher levels of inflammatory markers were associated with lesser amounts of coronary artery disease.

The Tsimane are an indigenous population that has maintained its traditional preindustrial lifestyle. At the population level, the Tsimane have an extremely low prevalence of obesity and coronary artery disease and thereby prove that obesity was a very uncommon phenotype prior to the emergence of our modern culture.

During our long evolutionary history, food scarcity would have been a much more frequent occurrence than food abundance. This evolutionary pressure would have led to selection of phenotypes that favored energy storage. The three evolutionary hypotheses discussed in the previous section outline genetic landscapes that could account for our physiological bias towards energy storage during times of food scarcity. Despite fluctuations in food availability, human populations prior to the introduction of agriculture had a very low prevalence of obesity. In preindustrial populations food intake generally matched physiological needs. By contrast, in our modern culture, food intake has become disconnected from physiological needs. Over the past 50 to 75 years excess food intake has become the norm and excess food intake is a primary factor promoting obesity. As already discussed, this excess food intake has occurred in the context of a physiological bias toward energy storage. I do not discount that our modern culture is characterized by a sedentary lifestyle and reduced physical activity but at a global level obesity prevalence correlates with trends in food consumption.

Modern Trends in Food Consumption

Kearney (2010) looked at global food consumption trends and the drivers of those trends. Kearney (2010) used food balance sheets which are country wide accounts of the supply and use of foods which are prepared by the Food and Agriculture Organization of the United Nations. Another source of data was individual dietary surveys done within countries.

Between 1969 and 2001 food consumption (kcal per person per day) increased globally (15.5%), in developing countries (25.7%) and in industrial countries (13.1%). Changes in food consumption patterns also occur when developing countries transition from traditional diets high in cereals, grains, vegetables and fibre to a Western type diet high in fat, sugar, oils and meats. These changes in food consumption have been referred to as the nutrition transition and this transition is associated with the emergence of chronic non-infectious degenerative diseases. Kearney (2010) looked at the various factors that drive food consumption. These included; income, urbanization, transnational food corporations, food industry marketing and consumer attitudes and behaviors. Kearney (2010) pointed out that the spread of obesity, particularly among lower and middle income groups, has occurred in parallel with the globalization of food systems and the expansion of transnational food corporations.

The relationship between food consumption and obesity is a very complex issue and there is an extensive literature on this topic. I have only touched the surface in this section. Energy dense diets are generally poor in micronutrients and so individuals who are obese can also be under nourished in terms of micronutrients. My point is that the current epidemic of obesity is being fueled by the consumption of excess calories and the factors that are driving consumption of excess calories are cultural.

In the next sections, I examine the influence of fast food outlets and transnational food corporations in the increasing prevalence of obesity.

Fast Food Outlets

Fast food outlets can be considered part of the urban food environment and the question posed is whether there is an association between fast food restaurant density and body mass index. Hollands et al., (2014) addressed this question using data from the Canadian Community Health Survey. The data set included adults between 18-65 years residing in one of Canada's ten provinces (n = 89,733). Neighbourhood socio-demographic variables were obtained from the 2006 Canadian census. The density of fast food, full-service and non-chain restaurants per 10,000 individuals in forward sortation areas was calculated from a business agency registry data base.

Fast food restaurant density had a positive relationship with BMI whereas full-service and non-chain restaurant density had a negative association with BMI. These results were obtained after controlling for individual level lifestyle, socioeconomic and demographic factors as well as neighbourhood level socioeconomic variables. These relationships were primarily found in Canada's major urban centres. As an example, for females of height 1.67 metres, a mean difference of 1.14 kg in weight was estimated between forward sortation areas that differed by 10 fast food restaurants per 10,000 population. This study supports the contention that a high density of fast food restaurants in an urban environment is associated with unhealthy eating behaviors as attested to by the positive relationship between BMI and fast food restaurant density. Density of fast food restaurants would be a component of the driver of food consumption that Kearney (2010) referred to as urbanization.

Murphy et al. (2018) investigated associations between food outlet access and BMI across urban growth and urban established areas of Melbourne Australia. The sample consisted of 3,141 respondents from the Melbourne metropolitan area drawn from a data set collected for the preventative health survey of 2012/2013. Of the 3,141 respondents, 1,648 resided in six established area municipalities in the more central part of Melbourne and 1,493 resided in six urban growth area municipalities on the fringe. A number of individual level and behavioral covariates were collected including frequency of fast food intake. The outcome variable was BMI and the exposure variables were supermarket and fast food chain access. Supermarket density and proximity were not associated with BMI for any access measures (walking/car/public transport) across established and urban growth areas. Fast food chain density within 800 metres and 1000 metres was associated with a higher BMI for respondents in established areas; for each additional fast food chain outlet, mean BMI increased by 0.20 kg/m2 and 0.27 kg/m2 for 800 and 1000 metre distances respectively. In contrast, fast food chain density was associated with a lower BMI for respondents in growth area municipalities within 800 metres and 1600 metres. The investigators had several possible explanations as to why the relationship between BMI and fast food chain density differed between respondents in established urban areas and respondents in urban growth areas. This study supports the major findings of Hollands et al. (2014) that a high urban density of fast food outlets promotes unhealthy eating behaviors, presumably a high caloric intake, which is associated with an increase in BMI.

Influence of a Transnational Food Corporation on Public Health Policies

Greenhalgh (2019 a, b) recently described how the transnational food corporation Coca-Cola influenced obesity science and policy in China on a national level. The sequence of events started in 1978 when Alex Malaspina, a senior Coca-Cola vice president founded the International Life Sciences Institute (ILSI) as a vehicle to disseminate science directed at improving human health and wellbeing. In 1993, Chen Chunming became the founding president of ILSI-China. ILSI has become a worldwide organization with seventeen branches including the one in China. Previously (1983) Chen Chunming had been the founding president of the Chinese Academy of Preventative Medicine, a division of the Ministry of Health. By 1997, seventeen companies supported ISLI-China and by 2015 this number had grown to thirty eight. These companies were predominantly food industry multinationals. ISLI-China's activities included newsletters and conferences.

In 1999, ISLI-China asked its affiliates to put obesity on their agenda and ISLI-China established itself as China's leading authority on obesity. ISLI-China created China specific BMI thresholds to define obesity and developed guidelines for the prevention and management of obesity. These guidelines were issued in the name of the Ministry of Health. Between 1999 and 2015, the focus of anti-obesity efforts shifted noticeably from nutritional strategies towards exercise base strategies. This change in focus was particularly evident after 2003. From 2010 to 2015, 60% of ISLI-China sponsored obesity efforts focused primarily on exercise as the primary strategy to manage the obesity epidemic.

Between 2004 and 2015, ISLI-China sponsored nine conferences and workshops on obesity. Six of the conferences were international and half of the invited experts were either exercise scientists or emphasized physical activity in their obesity research. These conferences promoted the notion that physical fitness was the most important strategy for combating obesity. Two of the speakers, who were invited most frequently, had received funding from Coca-Cola. In 2015, the New York Times reported that Coca-Cola had paid leading exercise focused scientists to establish a Global Energy Balance Network to promote the concept that inactivity not poor diet was the root cause of obesity.

In the decade after Coca-Cola launched its obesity campaign, the focus of China's obesity science and interventions changed markedly from diet to physical activity.

There are links between Coca-Cola and other exercise initiatives in China; Happy 10 Minutes, a school exercise program and Healthy Lifestyles for All Campaign.

Quoting from Greenhalgh (2019 b); "This is the first study to empirically substantiate not just the efforts, but also the impact of the soda industry on the obesity science and policy of any nation. Though that impact cannot be measured with quantitative precision, China's policies aligned well with Coke's position as transmitted through ISLI-China."

As noted, in indigenous populations such as the Tsimane, food intake generally matched physiological needs. Over the past 50 to 75 years food intake has become disconnected from physiological needs and excessive food intake is now considered the root cause of the current obesity epidemic. How does food intake become disconnected from physiological needs? To address this question, I review the science of the flavor system in the human brain. The brain flavor system is one of the primary determinants of eating behaviors.

Science of Flavor

It is difficult to give a good definition as to what constitutes the flavor of a food. Taste is the most obvious component but flavor is a multisensory construct involving visual, touch (by the tongue) and odor sensory stimuli. There is also a connection between language and flavors; words are used to communicate what are desirable or undesirable flavors. A seminal paper on this topic was written by Shepherd in 2006. In fact, Shepherd imagined a new discipline of science termed "neurogastronomy" which was a combination of the biochemistry of food preparation and the molecular biology of the olfactory and brain flavor systems.

Odor stimulation of olfactory sensory cells in the nose involves odor molecules interacting with olfactory sensory receptor proteins. Humans have about 350 genes that code for these proteins. The axons of sensory neurons project to the olfactory bulb where they converge onto modules known as glomeruli. Different odor molecules are represented by different spatial patterns of activity in the olfactory bulb. These activity patterns create odor images or odor maps. According to Shepherd (2006) this odor sensory system is analogous to the complex visual sensory system that recognizes human faces. (Shepherd's paper clearly predated our current understanding of the details underlying the visual code by which we recognize facial patterns that I described in a previous section in this *Chapter*.)

Orthonasal stimulation refers to the sniffing in through the external nares of odor molecules which activate the sensory cells in the olfactory epithelium. Signals are transmitted to the olfactory bulb and then on to the olfactory cortex in the orbital part of the prefrontal cortex.

Retronasal stimulation occurs during food ingestion. Volatile molecules released from food in the oropharynx are pumped by muscular action up through the nasopharynx to the olfactory epithelium. Because these volatile molecules arise from food in the mouth they are referred to the mouth i.e., they are perceived as if they were sensed within the mouth and are judged to be part of the taste of food. Thus, although a large part of flavor is due to smell, it is attributed to taste.

Taste is the most obvious component of food flavor and receptor cells that respond to the five basic tastes (sweet, salty, sour, bitter and umami) are assembled into taste buds which are distributed across different papillae of the tongue and palate epithelium. Taste signals ascend from the brainstem to the hypothalamus and from there to the thalamus and then to the primary taste cortex.

Shepherd (2006) paints a complex picture of the many sensory modalities that feed into the brain flavor system and the links between the brain flavor system and brain regions that are activated by food cravings. These are the same brain regions that are activated by alcohol and drug addiction. The key parts of this picture are as follows. The sensory modalities that feed into the brain flavor system include; vision (color and shape), somatosensory (temperature, touch, texture), taste (bitter, salty, sour, sweet and umami plus retronasal odor stimulation), and smell. The brain regions comprising the flavor system include; neocortex, hippocampus, olfactory and limbic systems, hypothalamus and the amygdala systems. The amygdala systems link the flavor system to emotion, motivation and craving circuits.

Quoting from Shepherd (2006); "Flavor perception is one of the most complex of human behaviors. It involves almost all of the senses, particularly the sense of smell, which is involved through odor images generated in the olfactory pathway. In the human brain, the perceptual systems are closely linked to systems for learning, memory, emotion and language, so distributed neural mechanisms contribute to food preference and food cravings. Greater recognition of the role of the brain's flavor system and its connection with eating behavior is needed for a deeper understanding of why people eat what they do, and to generate better recommendations about diet and nutrition."

In summary, an individual's food flavor images are a primary determinant of that individual's eating behaviors and food cravings. Since food flavor images are constructed from the inputs of multiple sensory modalities, these sensory modalities become targets that can be manipulated with a view to modifying eating behaviors. Such a strategy has been used by the food industry to promote the eating, even to excess, of so called fast foods which are generally calorie dense but of poor nutritional value.

There is very good evidence that our current epidemic of obesity and its allied metabolic disorder type 2 diabetes is due to excessive food intake that exceeds physiological needs and that generally involves calorie dense food that is of poor nutritional value. It would be an oversimplification to say that this epidemic at the population level is due to collective individual poor food choices; the population level excessive food intake underlying this epidemic is culturally driven. The food industry has promulgated cultural practices that involve how foods are packaged, how foods are advertised and marketed and what specific words are used to describe foods to create attractive and pleasurable flavor images of these foods. Such pleasurable flavor images entice individuals to eat those foods even to excess. In addition so called fast food is enriched with fat, sugar and salt, a particularly flavorful combination that is not found in natural food. There is evidence that the density of fast food outlets in our urban space creates a food environment that correlates in a positive direction with population body mass index. Finally a transnational food corporation has been successful in changing the obesity prevention health policies of a country from a nutrionally based strategy to an exercise based strategy. These cultural practices have all been instituted for economic gain.

Sleep Disorders

In *chapter 1*, I discussed sleep patterns across species including humans. For humans, the sleep patterns of ancestral pre-industrial populations have been gauged by extrapolating from the measured sleep characteristics of three surviving pre-industrial societies (see *Chapter 1*). A telling observation was that these surviving pre-industrial societies did not have a word for insomnia. In this section the focus will be on the cultural origin of present day sleep disorders and the apparent consequences of those disorders. In *Chapter 1*, I reviewed a study that measured the impact of artificial light on sleep patterns. This study compared two indigenous groups, one with and one without access to electric light. The group with access to electric light had shorter sleep duration in both winter and summer compared to the "no electric light access" group. The difference in sleep duration was due to later bedtimes and sleep onsets in the group with access to artificial light. Sleep offsets and rise times were the same for both groups. This study illustrates that even a simple cultural device, electric light, can be associated with measurable effects on sleep patterns. The effects of more complex cultural practices are discussed in the following sections.

Population Burden of Sleep Disorders

There have been a number of surveys at the population level of unhealthy sleep behaviors, but I will only reference one. The Centers for Disease Control and Prevention (CDC) in the United States sponsors a Behavioral Risk factor Surveillance System (BRFSS) that is a state-based random- digit- dialed telephone survey of the noninstitutionalized U.S. civilian population aged eighteen years and older, conducted by state health departments in collaboration with CDC. In 2009 a sleep module was added to the BRFSS. In 2011, the CDC published the results of the 2009 survey which was based upon data from over 74,000 respondents across twelve states (McKnight-Eily et al., 2011; Wheaton et al., 2011). I summarize only the overall results although the data were analyzed in terms of a number of sociodemographic variables; age, gender, employment status, educational level, marital status, state of residence. Thirty-five percent of respondents reported sleeping less than seven hours in a 24 hour period. Forty-eight percent reported snoring. Almost thirty-eight percent of respondents reported unintentionally falling asleep during the day at least one day in the preceding thirty days. Almost five percent of respondents reported nodding off or falling asleep while driving in the preceding thirty days. The results of the survey indicated that the percentage of certain sleep related behaviors differed according to the amount of sleep reported by respondents. For example, respondents were categorized as to whether they reported sleep duration of less than seven hours or seven or more hours in a 24 hour period. Snoring, unintentionally falling asleep during the day at least one day during the preceding thirty days and nodding off or falling asleep while driving during the preceding thirty days all had a higher prevalence in the respondent population sleeping less than seven hours in a 24 hour period than the population sleeping seven or more hours in a 24 hour period.

In the same 2011 publication, the authors stated that the percentage of U.S. adults reporting an average of less than seven hours of sleep per 24 hour period had substantially increased between 1985 and 2004 and they attributed this increase in part to broad societal changes including increase in technology use and shift work.

The results of this survey indicate that sleep deprivation is a widespread and relatively recent phenomenon in a developed country such as the United States. This finding is even more striking when put in the context that indigenous populations, as previously noted, have no word for insomnia.

The data for sleep duration in this survey are self-reported and should be compared to the sleep period duration of 6.9 to 8.5 hours reported by Yetsin et al., (2015; see *Chapter 1.*) for living indigenous populations. Hence by comparison to pre-industrial populations, a sleep period duration of less than 7 hours should be considered as constituting sleep deprivation. What follows are examples of cultural induced sleep disorders.

Culture and Sleep Disorders

Example 1: Artificial Light

Perhaps the most significant cultural innovation that affected sleep patterns was the commercialization of the incandescent light bulb at the end of the nineteenth century (Chepesiuk, 2009). This innovation prolonged the length of the work day and provided more time for recreational activities. However there has been a biological cost to development of artificial light. As discussed in *Chapter 1* and in this section on *Sleep disorders*, the introduction of electric light into an indigenous population resulted in shorter sleep duration by almost an hour. Artificial light has also made possible shift work which results in disruption of the circadian rhythm and alterations in sleep patterns.

In addition, the extensive use of artificial lighting in our urban centers has led to a phenomenon known as nighttime light pollution. As noted by Chepesiuk (2009) the sky glow from Los Angeles is visible from an airplane 200 miles away. Singapore is one of the most light polluted regions on the globe. At the population level, nighttime light pollution due to artificial light is one of the defining characteristics of life in the modern world (Chepesiuk, 2009).

The health effects of light pollution on humans are not well understood. Light pollution in urban areas very likely disrupts the circadian rhythm and sleep patterns of residents in that urban environment and through these effects light pollution could pose a serious health risk. As described by Chepesiuk (2009), across 147 communities in Israel, there was a significant correlation between the level of nighttime artificial light and the distribution of breast cancer.

Example 2: Sleep and Memory

As noted in *Chapter 1*, there is still no consensus as to the core function of sleep i.e., the core ancestral function responsible for its evolutionary emergence is unknown (Rolls et al., 2011). One proposal is that sleep supports memory consolidation and Rolls et al., (2011) tested this construct experimentally in a mouse model.

Hypocretin/orexin (Hcrt) producing neurons in the lateral hypothalamus regulate sleep-wake transitions by setting a threshold for arousals. Rolls et al., (2011) used a viral vector to insert the gene for the light sensitive cation channel channelrhodopsin-2 (ChR2) into Hcrt neurons in the mouse lateral hypothalamus. After three weeks, Hcrt neurons transduced with the virus achieved sufficient expression of channelrhodopsin-2. An optical fiber inserted into the brain was used to deliver light pulses to the lateral hypothalamus. Light pulses activate the transduced Hcrt neurons through their effects on the structure of the expressed light sensitive channelrhodopsin-2 cation channel. Each stimulus comprised 10 seconds of light pulses and stimulations were delivered every 30 or 60 seconds. Light stimulus activation of Hcrt neurons increased the probability of transition from a sleep state to wakefulness.

The investigators made the following observations with both the 30 and 60 seconds stimulation protocols as compared to controls. Both protocols increased the number of transitions from rapid eye movement (REM) and non-rapid eye movement (NREM) sleep to wakefulness compared to controls. The increased number of transitions to wakefulness was accompanied by a decrease in mean duration of NREM sleep episodes but no change in the mean duration of REM sleep episodes. Stimulation also resulted in a decrease in the mean duration of wake episodes. For mice treated with the 60 seconds stimulation protocol, despite the fragmented sleep architecture, the percentage of total time spent in wakefulness, NREM and REM sleep was the same as controls. This observation was not true for the 30 seconds stimulation protocol; percentage of total time in wakefulness increased and percentage of total time in NREM sleep decreased. Hence, the 60 seconds protocol did not change the overall amount of sleep or the relative composition of sleep i.e., the 60 seconds stimulation protocol caused a change in sleep architecture notably fragmentation.

Rolls et al., (2011) used the 60 seconds stimulation protocol to assess the effects of fragmented sleep on the process of memory consolidation in this mouse model. Memory consolidation was tested using the Novel Object recognition Task. Briefly, at the training session, control mice and mice transduced with ChR2 were allowed to explore an open arena containing two similar objects. The mice usually explore the two objects equally. At the end of this session, the ChR2 mice were stimulated for four hours during their resting phase using the 60 seconds stimulation protocol. Twenty four hours later, control and ChR2 mice were re-examined in the same arena but with one of the previously encountered objects replaced by a novel one. If the mouse spends more time during this testing session with the novel object, it is considered an indication that the mouse remembered the other familiar object. The stimulated ChR2 mice did not explore the novel object longer than the familiar one. Controls spent 65% of time exploring the novel object while ChR2 stimulated mice spent about 50% of time exploring the novel object. The investigators concluded that fragmentation or loss of sleep continuity impaired memory consolidation.

Since the stimulation protocols did not affect REM sleep, the investigators proposed that sleep continuity independent of sleep amount is critical for memory consolidation in mice and more specifically, that a minimum length of continuous NREM sleep was necessary for memory consolidation.

The experimental observations of Rolls et al., (2011) are consistent with the functions of sleep spindles (Schonauer and Pohlchen, 2018). Sleep spindles are isolated bursts of oscillatory neural activity observed during NREM but not REM sleep. The spindle rhythm stems from coordinated activity within three brain regions; thalamus, thalamic-reticular nucleus and neocortex. Sleep spindles have been found in all mammals but not in birds. Sleep spindles occur throughout the night and across different sleep stages. Sleep spindles are partly responsible for sensory shutdown during sleep. Brain responses to external stimuli are diminished and it is more difficult to wake someone while sleep spindles are generated. Humans retained information better when we get the opportunity to sleep after learning. Repeated activation of the neural ensembles that constitute a memory seems to be crucial to forming lasting memories i.e., memory consolidation. The evidence is that sleep spindles during NREM sleep play a critical role in the process of memory consolidation (Cairney et al., 2018).

The experimental observations of Rolls et al., (2011) and the observations regarding the functional role of sleep spindles (Cairney et al. 2018; Schonauer and Pohlchen, 2018) indicate that a minimal unit of uninterrupted sleep, particularly NREM sleep, is crucial for memory consolidation. Sleep fragmentation is detrimental to memory consolidation. *The corollary would be that artificial light sources, be it electric light bulbs or light emitting devices, that change sleep architecture would impair the process of memory consolidation.*

Example 3: Media Screen Time and Sleep Patterns

The following are two studies in which investigators examined the effects of light emitting devices and media screen time on sleep patterns.

Chang et al., (2015) looked at the effects of using a light-emitting e-reader at night on sleep patterns. The experimental design was as follows. Twelve healthy young adults (mean age 24.9 years, half female) completed two protocols in a crossover design. One protocol consisted of reading a light-emitting e-reader (LE-e-book) in very dim room light for four hours before bedtime for five consecutive evenings. The second protocol was similar except a printed book (print-book) read using reflected light in the same very dim room light was substituted for the e-reader. The investigators measured sleep patterns, sleep composition and plasma melatonin levels. Chang et al., (2015) made the following observations.

Evening levels of melatonin were suppressed by a mean of 55% during the LE-e-book protocol compared to the print-book protocol. Dim light onset of melatonin secretion occurred 90 minutes later on the day following the LE-e-book protocol compared to the print-book protocol. Sleep latency (time interval between lights out and sleep onset) was longer and REM sleep was of shorter duration with the LE-e-book protocol. Total sleep duration, sleep efficiency and duration of NREM sleep were comparable for both protocols. Participants rated themselves as being sleepier the morning after reading using the light-emitting e-book.

In summary, reading a light-emitting e-book prior to bedtime changed the circadian timing of melatonin secretion, altered sleep composition (less REM sleep) and was associated with a feeling of sleepiness the next morning.

Twenge et al. (2017) looked at self-reported sleep duration in adolescents and its correlation with media screen time. These investigators used two large surveys administered in the United States; the Monitoring the Future (MtF) survey and the Youth Risk Behavior Surveillance System (YRBSS). The MtF survey samples 8th, 10th and 12th graders and the investigators collected data from 1991 to 2015. The YRBSS surveys 9th, 10th, 11th and 12th graders and data were collected for the period 1991 to 2015. Both surveys contained questions as to how much sleep the respondents got.

By 2015 more than 40% of adolescents reported getting less than seven hours of sleep on most nights across both datasets. In 1991, only 26% of participants reported insufficient sleep of less than seven hours. The data also showed that the number of adolescents getting insufficient sleep increased abruptly between 2011 and 2013. The investigators examined for temporal trends in different activities over the time period 2009 to 2015 that correlated with this increase in the prevalence of short sleep duration of less than seven hours. Three activities were associated with increased odds of short sleep duration and showed an increase in usage between 2009 and 2015; electronic device use, social media use, and internet news consumption. TV watching actually decreased over this same time period. The investigators further analyzed the data for electronic device use. Use of electronic devices for more than one hour per day was positively correlated with sleep duration of less than seven hours. Thirty five percent of teens using electronic devices for one hour per day slept less than seven hours. This percentage increased to 52% for teens using electronic devices for five or more hours per day.

The investigators concluded that between 2009 and 2015, the most plausible factor accounting for the increase in short sleep duration reported by participating adolescents was the increase in new media screen time activities.

In summary, together these studies by Chang et al. (2015) and Twenge et al. (2017) highlight the deleterious effects that new media screen time can have on sleep patterns. These two studies combined underscore that excessive use of new electronic media devices is associated with shorter sleep duration, altered circadian timing of melatonin secretion and changes in sleep composition.

Example 4: Sleep and Cardiac and Metabolic Variables

There have been a number of studies linking sleep disorders to cardiovascular and metabolic disorders and several review articles have summarized the results of these studies.

Spiegel et al., (2009) reviewed the effects of short sleep duration and poor quality sleep on glucose metabolism and risk of obesity. Poor quality sleep referred to suppression of NREM sleep. In human subjects, both short duration and poor quality sleep decreased glucose tolerance (rate of decrease of glucose levels after an intravenous load) partly due to reduced insulin sensitivity. Reduced sleep duration has been associated with decreased plasma levels of leptin, a satiety hormone, and increased plasma levels of ghrelin, an appetite stimulating hormone. The changes in glucose handling and the changes in leptin and ghrelin levels associated with short duration and/or poor quality sleep may partly explain the epidemiological evidence linking short duration and/or poor quality sleep to the risk of obesity and type 2 diabetes (Spiegel et al., 2009).

Tobaldini et al., (2018) reviewed the evidence that short sleep duration was a risk for cardiovascular disorders such as coronary artery disease, hypertension and arrhythmias. The potential links between short sleep duration and adverse cardiovascular outcomes are all indirect and involve alterations in autonomic nervous system function, altered glucose regulation and altered endothelial function to name a few. This review highlighted the potential extent of the health consequence of short sleep duration.

Recently, McAlpine et al., (2019) presented experimental evidence for a link between sleep fragmentation and atherosclerosis. These investigators used a mouse model genetically engineered to be atherosclerotic prone (Apoe -/- mice). A high fat diet in these mice accelerates the development of atherosclerotic lesions. In one group of animals sleep fragmentation (SF) was induced by moving a bar intermittently across the bottom of the animals' cages during their sleep period. A second group of animals, not subjected to the sleep fragmentation protocol, served as controls (C). Both groups were fed a high fat diet. After eight weeks, SF mice showed larger atherosclerotic lesions than controls. In addition, aortas from SF mice contained more neutrophils, monocytes and macrophages than the aortas from C mice. The investigators explored the steps that led from sleep fragmentation to accelerated atherosclerotic lesions.

SF mice showed increased bone marrow hematopoietic stem cells and other progenitor subsets i.e., sleep fragmentation promoted myelopoiesis. The investigators focused on the hypothalamus and the expression of sleep regulating proteins. They found that sleep fragmentation, compared to controls, decreased the expression of hypothalamic hypocretin/orexin (Hcrt), a neuropeptide that regulates sleep-wake transitions. Bone marrow from mice that lack hypocretin (Hcrt -/-) have more hematopoietic progenitors along with increased proliferation of stem cells. Hence the increased hematopoiesis in SF mice was most likely due to decreased hypothalamic production of hypocretin since hypothalamic produced hypocretin can enter the circulation and affect hematopoiesis in the distal bone marrow.

McAlpine et al., (2019) identified a Hcrt receptor on bone marrow pre-neutrophils. Pre-neutrophils produce colony stimulating factor-1 (CSF1), which promotes bone marrow myeloid-biased hematopoiesis. However, hypocretin through its interaction with the Hcrt receptor acts to reduce the production of CSF1 by pre-neutrophils. Since sleep fragmentation is associated with decreased hypothalamic expression of Hcrt, under these circumstances pre-neutrophils would not be constrained in their production of CSF1.

In summary, sleep fragmentation reduced hypothalamic production of hypocretin which allowed increased myelopoiesis via greater pre-neutrophil production of CSF1. The increased production of neutrophils and monocytes was associated with migration of these cells to arterial walls. There monocytes developed into macrophages and macrophages and to a lesser extent neutrophils promoted the formation of atherosclerotic plaques.

At the population level, the emergence of sleep disorders can be dated to the commercialization of artificial light in the latter part of the nineteenth century. Artificial light has become so extensive in some urban areas that residents are exposed to a constant dim glow all night. Artificial light has had a profound effect on our sleeping patterns. In addition over the past fifty to sixty years personal electronic devices including computer, television, tablets, smart phones and e-readers have been developed.

These personal electronic devices have become ubiquitous and are used predominantly for social communication and transfer of information. The use of these personal electronic devices has also had a profound effect on sleeping patterns adding to the effects of an environment suffused with artificial light. The sleep changes associated with the use of personal electronic devices and the ever presence of artificial light include; shorter duration of sleep, changes in sleep architecture such as reduction of REM sleep, fragmentation of sleep continuity particularly in NREM sleep and alterations in the circadian timing of melatonin secretion. What have been the consequences of these changes in sleep patterns? It is too early to know whether the widespread use of electronic devices and the ever presence of artificial light will select out certain gene alleles. Could there be epigenetic effects? I am not aware of any data with regard to this possibility. However there is good evidence that certain changes in sleep architecture such as fragmentation in NREM sleep impair the process of memory consolidation. The links between short sleep duration and altered sleep composition to obesity, type 2 diabetes, cancer and cardiovascular disorders are all indirect and mainly epidemiological. However, as noted in the previous section, there are experimental data linking sleep fragmentation to atherosclerosis in a mouse model. I think it is safe to say that artificial light and personal electronic devices, recent cultural innovations, have come with a significant biological cost. The full extent of that biological cost is yet to be known.

CONCLUSION

The title of this chapter contains the word *Aging* which begs the question as to how the cultural driven phenotypic changes discussed in this chapter have shaped human aging. At the species level the aging process is coded in a developmental program specific to that species. Aging begins at the time of conception when this developmental program is triggered. Hence, aging should not be viewed as a specific stage in an organism's life cycle. Within a species, there are considerable variations in the aging process between individuals. These variations are due to the plasticity of the developmental program as well as its inherent stochasticity. At the level of the species, the aging trajectory is characterized in terms of age-specific measures of fertility and survival probability. As discussed in *Chapter 1*, each species has its own unique aging trajectory underwritten by its own unique developmental program. Another example of this uniqueness is contained in a report by Callier (2019) who recently reviewed the evolutionary strategies that long-lived large-bodied animals employed to resist cancer i.e., Peto's Paradox. These strategies appear to be species-specific consistent with the uniqueness of each species developmental program. At the level of the individual, as compared to the species, we generally view the aging phenotype as much richer and more nuanced than simply survival and reproduction.

Since divergence of the human lineage from its common ancestor with bonobo and chimpanzee, culture has played a critical role in shaping the evolutionary course of the human lineage. Culture has deep evolutionary roots as discussed in the first section of this chapter and is not unique to humans. However, what does appear to be unique to the human lineage is cumulative culture. It is difficult to know when cumulative culture evolved but the first stone tools (Oldowan tools) are about two million years old and tool making is clearly a cumulative cultural activity i.e., the skills to make stone tools were passed down with modifications to subsequent generations. Cultural activities such as dairy farming, stone tool making, hybridization and migration out of Africa to distant parts of the globe resulted in significant phenotypic changes that were accompanied by selection for specific gene alleles. Since Homo sapiens emerged only 300,000 years ago, cultural activities such as stone tool making, which activity is at least two million years old, must have originated in archaic hominins prior to the appearance of Homo sapiens. Other cultural activities such as dairy farming and agriculture, migration out of Africa and hybridization with other hominin species directly involved Homo sapiens.

As discussed in *Chapter 1*, the evolution of Homo sapiens was accompanied by changes in the aging pattern. There was a trend of increased survivorship of older adults during this evolutionary course with the greatest increase in longevity occurring about 40,000 to 12,000 years ago. By about 35,000 years ago the modern human brain had evolved and the present aging pattern of Homo sapiens was established in hunter-gatherers approximately 10,000 to 12,000 years ago. This pattern was characterized by post-reproductive longevity in females, low adult mortality rates from maturity at age 15 years to age 40 years and thereafter an exponentially increasing mortality rate with a modal age of death of 72 years. The predominant causes of morbidity and mortality in hunter-gatherers were trauma, accidental or due to violence, and infectious diseases. Cultural innovations such as the ones discussed in this chapter have been an important driver in the evolution of this aging pattern. I would characterize cultural innovations such as tool making, global migrations, agriculture and dairy farming as utilitarian in nature.

There is no question that in modern times both the pace and nature of cultural innovations have changed. What is difficult is to define when this change in cultural innovations occurred. I would suggest the break point is the late nineteenth century with the invention of the telephone and the commercialization of artificial light. In England in the 1700s the predominant causes of death and morbidity were febrile illnesses. Over the past fifty to seventy five years there has been a significant change in the human aging pattern. As a species we are living longer but infectious diseases as the primary cause of morbidity and mortality have been replaced by chronic non-infectious diseases such as type 2 diabetes, obesity, sleep disorders and cardiovascular disorders. The emergence of these chronic non-infectious diseases is not genetically based. Our genome is not that different from that of hunter-gatherer populations (see discussion on the indigenous Tsimane of Bolivia in *Chapters 1, 3*). The emergence of these chronic non-infectious diseases has been driven by recent cultural innovations and activities. As discussed in *Chapter 2*, these non-infectious diseases should be viewed as variants of the modern human aging phenotype.

What is different about the nature of recent cultural innovations and activities? Many recent cultural innovations do have a utilitarian value. There are cars, trucks and airplanes to move people and goods from place A to place B. There are computers, machines and robots to perform jobs previously done by humans. But there is a subset of recent cultural innovations that may be considered to have an entertainment value. These innovations include hand held personal electronic devices which are used primarily for social communication and information transfer. In addition there are cultural activities directed at modifying human physiology primarily for economic gain. The two obvious examples are the tobacco industry which adjusted the nicotine content of cigarettes to make them addicting and the food industry which has manipulated the flavors of foods to promote their over consumption at a population level. As discussed in this chapter, these cultural innovations and practices have fueled the epidemic-like prevalence of obesity, metabolic disorders such as type 2 diabetes, ADHD and sleep disorders to name a few. These disorders are now part of our species aging phenotype.

There is one other cultural innovation that needs recognition and that is the process of urbanization. The introduction of plant and animal domestication plus agricultural practices gave humans access to a more stable food supply than available to hunter-gatherers. These cultural innovations made possible the process of urbanization. Today more than half of the world lives in urban environments and many of these urban centers contain more than ten million residents. (In 2017 there were thirty seven megacities defined as urban areas with more than ten million residents.) As I speculated in this *Chapter*, urbanization drove humans to evolve a more multidimensional theory of mind which enabled individuals to engage in both direct and indirect social interactions and economic exchanges in such large populations. In addition, urban populations had to define cultural norms with respect to what constituted "normal" human behavior. Individuals whose behavior fell outside the boundaries of these cultural norms were deemed to have a psychiatric disorder.

It is important to look at the changing role of culture in the evolutionary history of the human lineage. During the early part of the evolutionary course, archaic hominins inhabited natural ecosystems and evolution would have been driven by natural selection acting on phenotypic variants that were adaptive for the existing ecological conditions. With the emergence of cumulative culture at least two million years ago, culture itself came to play a progressively more important role in the evolutionary process. I would estimate that about 10,000 to 15,000 years ago at the onset of the Neolithic revolution, culture became the primary driver of human evolution. Now with more than half of the word's human population living in synthetic urban ecosystems, culture has become an even more dominant driver of human evolution. Since humans are the crafters of cultural innovations, this makes us to some extent the instrument of our own evolution.

Finally, one might argue that obesity, type 2 diabetes, cardiovascular disorders and sleep disorders are really lifestyle issues and reflect poor choices on the part of individuals. I would contend that this statement represents an oversimplification. I have presented evidence that recent cultural innovations and practices are the real culprit. As a corollary, we know that past cultural innovations such as tool making, agriculture, global migration to name a few significantly shaped the course of human evolution. It is much too early to determine how the course of human evolution will be shaped by recent cultural innovations that have occurred within the past one hundred years.

EPILOGUE

Present day human culture is enriched with technologies. In addition we as a species have a proclivity to use technology as a problem solving approach. A few examples will illustrate this point. Geoengineering or climate engineering has been advocated as a solution to the problem of climate change. In the area of medical care, there are a number of technologies that have been developed to solve specific problems. Cardiologists are now capable of threading catheters into coronary arteries and removing blockages. A stent can be inserted into the coronary artery to prevent the recurrence of an occlusion. For individuals who are obese, the technique of bariatric surgery is available to induce weight loss. These technologies solve specific problems but clearly do not address the underlying causative factors. As outlined in the *Introduction*, many countries are dealing with a growing population of aging individuals with a high proportion of the older population suffering from chronic non-infectious diseases. How societies manage this problem will be influenced by our understanding of the nature of the aging process, what constitutes a disease and the relationship between aging and diseases.

As described in the *Introduction*, the current view is that aging is the time-dependent accumulation of biological damage that occurs after attainment of reproductive maturity resulting from the diminished strength of natural selection. A number of dysregulated molecular processes have been identified and are considered to be responsible for the accumulated somatic damage. Within this framework it is difficult to disentangle "normal" aging and disease. Many researchers view aging as a major risk factor for chronic non-infectious diseases while other researchers have even proposed that aging itself be considered a disease (see *Introduction*). This current view of the aging process implies that correction of underlying dysregulated processes should result in disease cures and the abolition or at least mitigation of the aging phenotype. These expectations are unrealistic but unfortunately are congruent with our societal view that technology can solve "all" problems. It is also important to point out several shortcomings in studies designed to examine the molecular biology of aging. These studies usually use selected animal models and these animals are not studied in their natural ecological niches and ecosystems but rather in controlled laboratory settings. The multiple interactions between diverse species that characterize an ecosystem are not considered. In essence aging cannot be studied as an isolated phenotypic trait but must be understood within the broader context of the process of speciation.

In this book I have presented evidence for an alternative view of aging, its relationship to disease and the role of culture in shaping the aging process.

Chapter 1. Each species has a specific aging trajectory that is coded in that species unique developmental program. Hence, aging begins at conception and should not be viewed as a specific stage in a species lifecycle. Within a species, there is considerable between individual variations in the aging process due to the plastic nature of the developmental program and its inherent stochasticity. In essence aging is part of the fabric of life. For aging, I propose that the *core ancestral function* that led to the evolutionary emergence of this phenotype is the transfer of information/signaling and resources from aged organisms, both single and multicellular, to younger organisms, both single and multicellular, which leads to a behavioral change in the younger organisms. The aging phenotype, being part of a developmental program, cannot be abolished but it can be modified since developmental programs are plastic.

Chapter 2. Since aging shows extensive between individual variations, a human population will establish cultural norms which define the boundaries for what are considered normal functions (physiology) and behaviors. Functions and behaviors outside these boundaries are considered abnormal by that population and designated as a disease. Hence diseases are actually cultural constructs and in reality are simply extreme variants of the aging process.

Chapter 3. Although culture has deep evolutionary roots, cumulative culture is probably unique to the human lineage. Cumulative culture refers to the transmission of a cultural practice to subsequent generations with the inclusion in that transmission of any modifications made to that practice by each generation. Culture has always been an important driver of human evolution but as discussed in *Chapter 3*, over the past 100 to 150 years there has been a significant change in both the pace and nature of cultural innovations. Over this same time period there has occurred the emergence of chronic non-infectious diseases such as obesity, sleep disorders, type 2 diabetes, ADHD and cardiovascular disorders which over the past 50 to 75 years have greatly increased in prevalence at the population level. In addition culture has now become the dominant driving force for human evolution.

In summary, aging is not a disease and disease is a cultural construct used to define variants of the aging process.

My intent in writing this book was to develop a framework that defined the biology of the aging process, the nature of diseases and the relationship between the aging process and diseases. My intent was not to propose specific solutions to the demographic problem of an increasing aging population carrying a significant disease burden. However, on the basis of the framework developed in this book I would make the following suggestions.

1. The aging phenotype can be modified with both technological and pharmacological interventions but the extent of these modifications will be limited by the degree of plasticity of the human developmental program.

2. Appealing to individuals to make better food choices and to restrict their use of novel cultural innovations such as personal electronic devices will be of limited effectiveness. The ability of large corporate entities in the food and technology industries to control and manipulate consumer behaviors and purchases needs to be regulated. The current epidemic of chronic non-infectious diseases is predominantly due to the cultural practices of these industries as described in *Chapter 3.*
3. We as a species have to become aware that cultural innovations and practices are now the chief driver of our own evolution. For cultural innovations and practices introduced over the past 100 years it is still too early to know whether the phenotypic changes associated with these cultural innovations and practices will become genetically based. Do cultural innovations somehow have to be screened as to their evolutionary consequences? We are now the instrument of our own evolution and to me personally that is a frightening realization.

REFERENCES

Abbott, A. 2018. The face detective. *Nature* 564: 176-179.

Ackermann, R. R., Mackay, A. and M. L. Arnold. 2016. The hybrid origin of "modern" humans. *Evolutionary Biology* 43:1-11.

Alberts, S. C., Altmann, J., Brockman, D. K. et al. 2013. Reproductive aging patterns in primates reveal that humans are distinct. *PNAS* 110:13440-13445.

Arrizabalaga, J. 1999. Medical causes of death in preindustrial Europe: some historiographical considerations. *Journal of the History of Medicine* 54: 241-260.

Baker, R. J. and R. D. Bradley. 2006. Speciation in mammals and the genetic species concept. *Journal of Mammology* 87: 643-662.

Barry, C., Schmitz, M. T., Jiang, P. et al. 2017. Species-specific developmental timing is maintained by pluripotent stem cells ex utero. *Developmental Biology* 423: 101-110.

Barry, C., Schmitz, M. T., Jiang, P. et al. 2017. Species-specific developmental timing is maintained by pluripotent stem cells ex utero. *Developmental Biology* 423: 101-110.

Beall, C. M. 2006. Andean, Tibetan, and Ethiopian patterns of adaptation to high-altitude hypoxia. *Integrative and Comparative Biology* 46: 18-24.

Bertossa, R. C. 2011. Morphology and behaviour: functional links in development and evolution. *Philosophical Transactions of the Royal Society B Biological Sciences* 366: 2056-2068.

Beyens, I., Valkenburg, P. M. and J. T. Piotrowski. 2018. Screen media use and ADHD-related behaviors: four decades of research. *PNAS* 115:9875-9881.

Bhupathiraju, S. N. and F. B. Hu. 2016. Epidemiology of obesity and diabetes and their cardiovascular complications. *Circulation Research* 118: 1723-1735.

Blount, Z. D., Lenski, R. E. and J. B. Losos. 2018. Contingency and determinism in evolution: replaying life's tape. *Science* 362: 665-674.

Boyer, P. B. 2018. *Minds Make Societies - How Cognition Explains The World Humans Create.* Yale University Press, New Haven.

Bray, G. A. 1990. Obesity: historical development of scientific and cultural ideas. *International Journal of Obesity* 14: 909-926.

Brewer, N., Young, R. L. and E. Barnett. 2017. Measuring theory of mind in adults with autism spectrum disorder. *Journal of Autism and Developmental Disorders* 47: 1927-1941.

Bronikowski, A. M., Altmann, J., Brockman, D. K. et al. 2011. Aging in the natural world: Comparative data reveal similar mortality patterns across primates. *Science* 331: 1325-1328.

Brune, M. 2005. "Theory of mind" in schizophrenia: a review of the literature. *Scizophrenia Bulletin* 31: 21-42.

Buffenstein, R. 2005. The naked mole-rat: a new long-living model for human aging research. *Journal of Gerontology, Biological Sciences* 60A: 1369-1377.

Bulterijs, S., Hull, R. S., Bjork, V.C.E. et al. 2015. It is time to classify biological aging as a disease. *Frontiers in Genetics,* do1:10.3389/fgene.2015.00205.

Bush, J. O. 2019. Editorial: signaling pathways instruct the blueprint of life. *Developmental Biology* 447: 1-2.

Cairney, S. A., Guttesen, A. a. V., El Marj, N. et al. 2018. Memory consolidation is linked to spindle –mediated information processing during sleep. *Current Biology* 28: 948-954.

Callaway, E. 2017. Genome studies attract criticism. *Nature* 546: 463.

Callier, V. 2019. Solving Peto's paradox to better understand cancer. *PNAS* 116: 1825-1828.

Caspari, R. 2016. The evolution of grandparents. *Scientific American* 25: 80-85.

Caspari, R. and S-H. Lee. 2004. Older age becomes common late in human evolution. *PNAS* 101: 10895-10900.

Champagne, F. A., Francis, D. D., Mar, A. et al. 2003. Variations in maternal care in the rat as a mediating influence for the effects of environment on development. *Physiology and Behavior* 79: 359-371.

Chang, A-M., Aeschbach, D., Duffy, J. F. et al. 2015. Evening use of light-emitting eReaders negatively affects sleep, circadian timing, and next-morning alertness. *PNAS* 112: 1232-1237.

Chepesiuk, R. 2009. Missing the dark-health effects of light pollution. *Environmental health perspectives* 117: A20-A27.

Christakis, D. A., Ramirez, J. S. B., Ferguson, S. M. et al. 2018. How early media exposure may affect cognitive function: a review of results from observations in humans and experiments in mice. *PNAS* 115: 9851-9858.

Colvert, E., Rutter, M., Kreppner, J. et al. 2008. Do theory of mind and executive function deficits underlie the adverse outcomes associated with profound early deprivation?: Findings from the English and Romanian adoptees study. *Journal of Abnormal Child Psychology* 36: 1057-1068.

Cori, A., Bi, K., Luke, C. et al. 2018. The genetic basis of adaptation following plastic changes in coloration in a novel environment. *Current Biology* 28: 2970-2977.

Cox, L. S. and C. Redman. 2017. The role of cellular senescence in ageing of the placenta. *Placenta* 52: 139-145.

Creanza, N., Kolodny, O. and M. W. Feldman. 2017. Cultural evolutionary theory: how culture evolves and why it matters. *PNAS* 114: 7782-7789.

Croft, D. P., Brent, L. J. N., Franks, D. W. et al. 2015. The evolution of prolonged life after reproduction. *Trends in Ecology and Evolution* 30: 407-416.

Danchin, E., Nobel, S., Pocheville, A. et al. 2018. Cultural flies: conformist social learning in fruitflies predicts long-lasting mate-choice traditions. *Science* 362: 1025-1030.

DeLacy, M. 1999. Nosology, mortality, and disease theory in the eighteenth century. *Journal of the History of Medicine* 54:261-284.

De la Iglesia, H. O., Fernandez-Duque, E., Golombek, D. A. et al.2015. Access to electric light is associated with shorter sleep duration in a traditionally hunter-gatherer community. *Journal of Biological Rhythms* 30: 342-350.

De Queiroz, K. 2007. Species concepts and species delimitation. *Systematic Biology* 56: 879-886.

De Villiers, J. G. and P. A. de Villiers. 2014. The role of language in theory of mind development. *Topics in Language Disorders* 34:313-328.

Dong, X., Milholand, B. and J. Vijg. 2018. Evidence for a limit to human lifespan. *Nature* 538: 257-259.

Duda, P. and J. Zrzavy. 2013. Evolution of life history and behavior in Hominidae: towards phylogenetic reconstruction of the chimpanzee-human last common ancestor. *Journal of Human Evolution* 65: 424-446.

Dvash, J. and S. G. Shamay-Tsoory. 2014. Theory of mind and empathy as multidimensional constructs-neurological foundations. *Topics in Language Disorders* 34: 282-295.

Editorial. Screen time. How much is too much? An analysis tries to get to the bottom of a crucial question. *Nature* 565: 265-266.

Ellis, S., Franks, D. W., Nattrass, S. et al. 2018. Analysis of ovarian activity reveal repeated evolution of post-reproductive lifespans in toothed whales. *Scientific Reports* 8:12833DOI:10.1038/s41598-018-31047-8.

Espiritu, J. R. D. 2008. Aging-related sleep changes. *Clinics in Geriatric Medicine* 24: 1-14.

Fabrega, Jr., H. 1975. The need for an ethnomedical science. *Nature* 189: 969-975.

Frankopan, P. 2017. *The Silk Roads - A New History of the World.* Vintage Books, Division of Penguin Random House LLC, New York.

Fraser, H. B., Khaitovich, P., Plotkin, J. B. et al. 2005. Aging and gene expression in the primate brain. *PLOS Biology* 3: issue 9 e274.

Gandal, M. J., Zhang, P., Hadjimichael, E. et al. 2018. Transcriptome–wide isoform-level dysregulation in ASD, schizophrenia, and bipolar disorder. *Science* 362: 1265-1279.

Gibbons, A. 2017. Oldest members of our species discovered in Morocco. *Science* 356: 993-994.

Goldman-Wohl, D. and S. Yagel. 2014. United we stand not dividing: the syncytiotrophoblast and cell senescence. *Placenta* 35: 341-344.

Greenbaum, G., Friesem, D. E., Hovers, E. et al. 2018. Was inter-population connectivity of Neanderthals and modern humans the driver of the Upper Paleolithic transition rather than its product? *Quaternary Science Reviews* doi.org/10.1016/j.quascirev.2018.12.011.

Greenhalgh, S. 2019 (a). Makin China safe for coke: how Coca-Cola shaped obesity science and policy in China. *British Medical Journal* 364:k5050doi:10.1136/bmj.k5050 (published 9 January 2019).

Greenhalgh, S. 2019 (b). Soda industry influence on obesity science and policy. *Journal of Public Health Policy* doi.org/10.1057/s41271-018-00158-x.

Guerrero-Bosagna, C. 2017. Evolution with no reason: a neutral view on epigenetic changes, genomic variability, and evolutionary novelty. *Bio Science* 67: 469-476.

Gurven, M. and H. Kaplan. 2007. Longevity among hunter-gatherers: a cross-cultural examination. *Population and Development Review* 33:321-365.

Hanaoka, M., Droma, Y., Basnyat, B. et al. 2012. Genetic variants in EPAS1 contribute to adaptation tp high-altitude hypoxia in Sherpas. *PLOS ONE* volume 7, issue 12, e50566.

Harris, S. E., Riggio, V., Evenden, L. et al. 2017. Age-related gene expression changes, and transcriptome wide association study of physical and cognitive aging traits, in Lothian Birth Cohort 1936. *Aging* 9: 2489-2503.

Harrison, S. E., Sozen, B., Christodoulou, N. et al. 2017. Assembly of embryonic and extraembryonic stem cells to mimic embryogenesis in vitro. *Science* 356: 153-164.

Hartenstein, V. and D. Jacobs. 2013. Developmental Plasticity, straight from the worm's mouth. *Cell* 155: 742-743.

Hashimoto, T., Horikawa, D. D., Saito, Y. et al. 2016. Extremotolerant tardigrade genome and improved radiotoleranve of human cultured cells by tardigrade-unique protein. *Nature Communications* doi:10.1038/ncomms12808.

Hatton, I. A., McCann, K. S., Fryxell, J. M. et al. 2015. The predator-prey power law: biomass scaling across terrestrial and aquatic biomes. *Science* 349 issue 6252, aac6284 doi: 10.1126/science.aac6284.

Healy, K. 2015. Eusociality but not fossoriality drives longevity in small mammals. *Proceedings of the Royal Society B* 282:20142917.doi.org/ 10.1098/rspb.2014.2917.

Helfrich-Forster, C. 2018. Sleep in insects. *Annual Review of Entomology* 63:69-86.

Herndon, C. N., Uiterloo, M., Uremaru, A. et al. 2009. Disease concepts and treatment by tribal healers of an Amazonian forest culture. *Journal of Ethnobiology and Ethnomedicine* 5:27, doi: 10.1186/1746-4269-5-27.

Hollands, S., Campbell, M. K., Gilliland, J. et al. 2014. Association between neighbourhood fast-food and full-service restaurant density and body mass index: a cross-sectional study of Canadian adults. *Canadian Public Health Association* 105 (3):e172-e178.

Horikawa, DE. D., Kunieda, T., Abe, W. et al. 2008. Establishment of a rearing system of the extremotolerant tardigrade Ramazzottius varieornatus: a new model animal for astrobiology. *Astrobiology* 8: 549-546.

Hu, H., Petousi, N., Glusman, G. et al. 2017. Evolutionary history of Tibetans inferred from whole-genome sequencing. *PLOS Genetics* doi.org/10.1371/journal.pgen.1006675.

Huerta-Sanchez, E., Jin, X., Asan. et al. 2014. Altitude adaptation in Tibetans caused by introgression of Denisovan-like DNA. *Nature* 512: 194-197.

Insel, T. R. 2010. Rethinking Schizophrenia. *Nature* 468: 187-193.

Irie, N. and Kuratani, S. 2014. The developmental hourglass model: a predictor of the basic body plan? *Development* 141: 4649-4655.

Jablonski, N. G. and G. Chaplin. 2017. The colors of humanity: the evolution of pigmentation in the human lineage. *Philosophical Transactions of the Royal Society B* 372:20160349.doi.org/101098/rstb.2016.0349.

Jaiswal, Y. S. and L. L. Williams. 2017. A glimpse of Ayurveda - The forgotten history and principles of Indian traditional medicine. *Journal of Traditional and Complementary Medicine* 7: 50-53.

Jamieson, L., Fauci, A. S., Kasper, D. L. et al. 2018. *Harrison's Principles of Internal Medicine,* 20th Edition. McGraw-Hill Education.

Jeong, C., Wilkin, S., Amgalantugs, T. et al. 2018. Bronze age population dynamics and the rise of dairy pastoralism on the eastern Eurasian steppe. *PNAS* 115: E11248-E11255.

Jesmer, B. R., Merkle, J. A., Goheen, J. R. et al. 2018. Is ungulate migration culturally transmitted? Evidence of social learning from translocated animals. *Science* 361: 10234-1025.

Joiner, W. J. 2016. Unravelling the evolutionary determinants of sleep. *Current Biology* 26: R1073-R1087.

Jones, O. R., Scheuerlein, A., Salguero-Gomez, R. et al. 2014. Diversity of ageing across the tree of life. *Nature* 505: 169-174.

Johnstone, R. A. and M. A. Cant. 2019. Evolution of menopause. *Current Biology* 29: R112-115.

Kampourakis, K. and F. Stern. 2018. Reconsidering the meaning of concepts in biology: why distinctions are so important. *BioEssays* DOI: 10.1002/bies.201800148.

Kaplan, H., Thompson, R. C., Trumble, B. C. et al. 2017. Coronary atherosclerosis in indigenous South American Tsimane: a cross-sectional cohort study. *Lancet* 389: 1730-1739.

Kalinka, A. T., Varga, K. M., Gerrard, D. T. et al. 2010. Gene expression divergence recapitulates the developmental hourglass model. *Nature* 468: 811-814.

Karels, T. J. and Boonstra, R. 2000. Concurrent density dependence and independence in populations of aectic ground squirrels. *Nature* 408: 460-463.

Kearney, J. 2010. Food consumption trends and drivers. *Philosophical Transactions of the Royal Society* B 365: 2793-2807.

Keji, C. and X. Hao. 2003. The integration of traditional Chinese medicine and Western medicine. *European Review* 11: 225-235

Kleinman, A., Eisenberg, L. and B. Good. 1978. Clinical lessons from anthropologic and cross-cultural research. *Annals of Internal Medicine* 88:251-258.

Koch, A., Brierley, C., Maslin, M. M. et al. 2019. Earth systems impacts of the European arrival and great dying in the Americas after 1492. *Quaternary Science Reviews* 207: 13-36.

Krabbendam, L. and J. V. Os. 2005. Schizophrenia and urbanicity: a major environmental influence - conditional on genetic risk. *Schizophrenia Bulletin* 31: 795-799.

Kremen, W. S., Beck, A., Elman, J. A. et al. 2019. Influence of young adult cognitive ability and additional education on later-life cognition. *PNAS* 10.1073/pnas.1811537116.

Krishnan, J. and N. Rohner. 2017. Cavefish and the basis for eye loss. *Philosophical Transactions of the Royal Society* B 372. 20150487 doi.org/10.1098/rstb.2015.0487.

Lahdenpera, M., Mar, K. U. and V. Lummaa. 2014. Reproductive cessation and post-reproductive lifespan in Asian elephants and pre-industrial humans. *Frontiers in Zoology* 11:54.

Laland, K. N., Odling-Smee, J. and S. Myles. 2010. How culture shaped the human geneome: bringing genetics and the human sciences together. *Nature Reviews Genetics* 11: 137-148.

Laland, K., Matthews, B. and M. W. Feldman. 2016. An introduction to niche construction theory. *Evolutionary Ecology* 30: 191-202.

Laland, K. 2018. How we became a different kind of animal-an evolved uniqueness. *Scientific American* 319: 33-39.

Lamichhaney, S., Han, F., Webster, M. T. et al. 2018. Rapid hybrid speciation in Darwin's finches. *Science* 359: 224-228.

Lee, P. C., Fishlock, V., Webber, C. E. et al. 2016. The reproductive advantages of a long life: longevity and senescence in wild female African elephants. *Behavioral Ecology and Sociobiology* 70: 337-345.

Lesku, J. A. and L. M. T. Ly. 2017. Sleep origins: restful jellyfish are sleeping jelly fish. *Current Biology* 27: R1060-R1062.

Levin, M., Anavy, L., Cole, A. G. et al. 2016. The mid-developmental transition and the evolution of animal body plans. *Nature* 531: 637-641.

Levis, N. A. and D. W. Pfennig. 2016. Evaluating "plasticity first" evolution in nature: key criteria and empirical approaches. *Trends in Ecology and Evolution* 31: 563-574.

Lin, M., Siford, R. L., Martin, A. R. et al. 2018. Rapid evolution of a skin-lightening allele in southern African KhoeSan. *PNAS* 115: 13324-13329.

Lopez-Otin, C., Blasco, M. A., Partridge, L. et al. 2013. The hallmarks of aging. *Cell* 153: 1194-1217.

Mallet, J. 2008. Hybridization, ecological races and the nature of species: empirical evidence for the ease of speciation. *Philosophical Transactions of the Royal Society* B363: 2971-2986.

Manoach, D. S. and R. Stickgold. 2016. Sleep: keeping one eye open. *Current Biology* 26: R360-R361.

Martin, A. R., Lin, M., Granka, J. M. et al. 2017. An unexpectantly complex architecture for skin pigmentation in Africans. *Cell* 171: 1340-1353.

McAlpine, C. S., Kiss, M. G., Rattik, S. et al. 2019. Sleep modulates haematopoiesis and protects against atherosclerosis. *Nature* 566: 383-387.

McBurney, S. H. 2012. Yin and Yang: the physical and the symbolic in Chinese medical practices. Totem: The University of Western Ontario *Journal of Anthropology* 20: Iss. 1, Article 5

McKnight-Eiloy, L. R., Liu, Y., Wheaton, A. G. et al. 2011. Unhealthy sleep-related behaviors- 12 States, 2009. *Morbidity and Mortality Weekly Report* (United States) 60: 233-238.

Meaney, M. J. and M. Szyf. 2005. Maternal care as a model for experience-dependent chromatin plasticity? *Trends in Neuroscience* 28: 456-463.

Menon, R., Behnia, F., Polettini, J. et al. 2016. Placental membrane aging and HMGB1 signaling associated with human parturition. *Aging 8:* 216-230.

Metzis, V., Steinhauser, S., Pakanavicius, E. et al. 2018. Nervous system regionalization entails axial allocation before neural differentiation. *Cell* 175: 1105-1118.

Meyer, D. E. 2018. From savannas to blue-phase LCD screens: prospects and perils for child development in the post-modern digital information age. *PNAS* 115: 9845-9850.

Mitchell, R. L. C. and A. H. Young. 2016. Theory of mind in bipolar disorder, with comparison to the impairments observed in schizophrenia. *Frontiers in Psychiatry* doi: 10.3389/fpsyt.201500188

Moore, A. 2013. On the state of scientific English and how to improve it-part 2. *Bioessays* 35: 497.

Munch, D. and G. V. Amdam. 2010. The curious case of aging plasticity in honey bees. F*EBS Letters* 584: 2496-2503.

Murphy, M., Badland, H., Jordan, H. et al. 2018. Local food environments, suburban development, and BMI: a fixed methods study. *International Journal of Environmental Research and Public Healthy* 15: 1392; doi: 10.3390/ijerph15071392

Narayanaswamy, V. 1981. Origin and development of Ayurveda. *Ancient Science of Life* 1: 1-7.

Nath, R. D., Bedbrook, C. N., Abrams, M. J. et al. 2017. The jellyfish Cassiopea exhibits a sleep-like state. *Current Biology* 27: 2984-2990.

Nelson, D. R. 2002. Current status of the Tardigrada: evolution and ecology. *Integrative and Comparative Biology* 42: 652-659.

Nelson, C. A. Fox, N. A. and C. H. Zeanah. 2014. Romania's Abandoned Children, Deprivation, *Brain Development, and the Struggle for Recovery.* Harvard University Press, Cambridge Massachusetts.

Nettle, D. and M. Bateson. 2015. Adaptive developmental plasticity: what is it, how can we recognize it and when can it evolve? *Proceedings of the Royal Society* B 28220151005.doi.org/10.1098/rspb.2015.1005.

Niebyl, P. H. 1071. Old age, fever, and the lamp metaphor. *Journal of the History of medicine and Allied Sciences* 26: 351368.

Neubauer, S., Hublin, J-J. and P. Gunz. 2018. The evolution of modern human brain shape. *Science Advances* 4: eaao5961.

Normile, D. 2018. Shock greets claim of CRISPR-edited babies. *Science* 362: 978—979.

Nunn, C. L., Samson, D. R. and A. D. Krystal. 2016. *Shining evolutionary light on human sleep and sleep disorders, Evolution, Medicine and Public Health.* doi:10.1093/emph/eow018.

Nussey, D. H., Froy, H., Lemaitre, J-F. et al. 2013. Senescence in natural populations of animals: widespread evidence and its implications for bio-gerontology. *Aging Research Reviews* 12: 214-225.

Nutton, V. 2018. Galen of Pergamum. *Encyclopedia Britannica,* www.britannica.com/biography/Galen-of-Pergamum.

Oates, A. C. 2011. What's all the noise about developmental stochasticity? *Development* 138: 601-607.

Ocampo, A., Reddy, P., Martinez-Redondo, P. et al. 2016. In vivo amelioration of age-associated hallmarks by partial reprogramming. *Cell* 167: 1719-1733.

Orlando, L. 2018. Late Bronze Age cultural origins of dairy pastoralism in Mongolia. *PNAS* 115: 12083-12085.

Partridge, L. 2018. Facing up to the global challenges of ageing. *Nature* 561: 45-56.

Patwardhan B., Warude, D. Pushpangadan, P. et al. 2005. Ayurveda and traditional Chinese medicine: a comparative overview. *Evidence-Based Complementary and Alternative Medicine* (eCAM); 2(4)465-473.

Peever, J. and P. M. Fuller. 2017. The biology of REM sleep. *Current Biology* 27: R1237-R1248.

Perry, B. W., Schield, D. R. and T. A. Castoe. 2018. Evolution: plasticity versus selection, or plasticity and selection? *Current Biology* 28: R1104-R1106.

Petersen, M C. and G. I. Shulman. 2018. Mechanisms of insulin action and insulin resistance. *Physiological Reviews* 98: 2133-2223.

Prud'homme, B. and N. Gompel. 2010. Genomic hourglass. *Nature* 468: 768-769.

Prufer, K., Munch, K., Hellmann, I. et al. 2012. The bonobo genome compared with the chimpanzee and human genomes. *Nature* 486: 527-531.

PsychENCODE Consortium. 2018. Revealing the brain's molecular architecture. *Science* 362: 1263.

Quesda, V., Freitas-Rodrguez, S., Miller, J. et al. 2018. Giant tortoise genomes provide insights into longevity and age-related disease. *Nature Ecology and Evolution.* doi.org/10.1038/s41559-018-0733-x.

Ragsdale, E. J., Muller, M. R., Rodelsperger, C. et al. 2013. A developmental switch coupled to the evolution of plasticity acts through a sulfatase. *Cell* 155: 922-933.

Rajagopalan, S. and E. O. Long. 2018. The landscape of early pregnancy. *Nature* 563: 337-338.

Rajarajan, P., Borrman, T., Liao, W. et al. 2018. Neuron-specific signatures in the chromosomal connectome associated with schizophrenic risk. *Science* 362. Issue 6420, eaat431. doi: 10.1126/ science.aat4311.

Reader, S. M., and K. Laland. 2002. Social intelligence, innovation, and enhanced brain size in primates. *PNAS* 99: 4436-4441.

Rivera-Mulia, J. C., Desprat, R., Trevilla-Garcia, C. et al. 2017. DNA replication timing alterations identify common markers between distinct progeroid diseases. *PNAS.* doi/10.1073/pnas.1711613114.

Roach, D. A. and J. R. Carey. 2014. Population biology of aging in the wild. *Annual Review of Ecology, Evolution and Systematics* 45: 421-443.

Rogers, A. R., Iltis, D. and S. Wooding. 2004. Genetic variation at the MC1R locus and the time since loss of human body hair. *Current Anthropology* 45: 105-108.

Rohner, N., Jarosz, D. F., Kowalko, J. E. et al. 2013. Cryptic variation in morphological evolution: HSP90as a capacitor for loss of eyes in cavefish. *Science* 342:1372-1375.

Rolls, A., Colas, D., Adamantidis, A. et al. 2011. Optogenetic disruption of sleep continuity impairs memory consolidation. *PNAS* 108: 13305-13310.

Row, J. R., Wilson, P. J. and D. L. Murray. 2014. Anatomy of a population cycle: the role of density dependence and demographic variability on numerical instability and periodicity. *Journal of Animal Ecology* 83: 800-812.

Sabatine, M. S., Giugliano, R. P., Keech, A. C. et al. 2017. Evolcumab and clinical outcomes in patients with cardiovascular disease. *New England Journal of Medicine* 376: 1713-1722.

Santini, F., Miglietta, M.P. and A. Faucci. 2012. Speciation: where are we now? An introduction to a special issue on speciation. *Evolutionary Biology* 39: 141-147.

Schonauer, M. and D. Pohlchen. 2016. Sleep spindles. *Current Biology* 28: R1129-R1130.

Scerri, E. M. L., Thomas, M. G., Manica, A. et al. 2018. Did our species evolve in subdivided populations across Africa, and why does it matter? *Trends in Ecology and Evolution 3*3: 582-594.

Sellayah, D., Cagampang, F. R. and R. D. Cox. 2014. On the evolutionary origins of obesity: a new hypothesis. *Endocrinology*155: 1573-1588.

Shapiro, B. J., Leducq, J-B. and J.Mallet. 2016. What is speciation? *PLOS Genetics* DOI: 10.1371/journal.pgen.1005860 March 31, 2016.

Shepherd, G.M. 2006. Smell images and the flavor system in the human brain. *Nature* 444:316-321.

Sima, J., Chakraborty, A., Dileep, V. et al. 2019. Identifying cis elements for spatiotemporal control of mammalian DNA replication. *Cell* 176: 816-830.

Singer, M. A. 2013. *Are Chronic Degenerative Diseases Part of the Ageing Process? Insights from Comparative Biology.* Nova Science Publishers, New York.

Singer, M. A. 2015. *Human Ageing, A Unique Experience. Implications for the Disease Concept.* World Scientific Publishing Company, Singapore.

Singer, M. A. 2016. The origins of aging: evidence that aging is an adaptive phenotype. *Current Aging Science* 9: 99-115.

Singer, M. A. 2018 a. Understanding Aging after Darwin. In *Aging, Exploring a Complex Phenomenon, ed*ited by Shamim I. Ahmad, 23-40. CRC Press, Taylor and Francis Group, Boca Raton.

Singer, M. A. 2018 b. The Origins of Aging: Multicellularity, Speciation, and Ecosystems. In *Aging, Exploring a Complex Phenomenon,* edited by Shamim I. Ahmad, 135-160. CRC Press, Taylor Francis Group, Boca Raton.

Sloan, D., Batista, R. A. and A. Loeb. 2017. The resilience of life to astrophysical events. *Scientific Reports* 7:P5419/ doi:10.1038/s41598-017-05796-x.

Slon, V., Mafessoni, F., Vernot, B. et al. 2018. The genome of the offspring of a Neanderthal mother and a Denisovan father. *Nature* 561: 113-116.

Spiegel, K., Tasali, E., Leproult, R. et al. 2009. Effects of poor and short sleep on glucose metabolism and obesity risk. *Nature Reviews Endocrinology* 5: 253-261.

Spikins, P., Needham, A., Tilley, L. et al. 2018. Calculated or caring? Neanderthal healthcare in social context. *World Archaeology,* DOI: 10.1080/00438243.2018.1433060.

Stanzione, C. and B. Schick. 2014. Environmental language factors in theory of mind development; evidence from children who are deaf/hard-of-hearing or who have specific language impairment. *Topics in Language Disorders* 34: 296-312.

Stout, D. 2011. Stone toolmaking and the evolution of human culture and cognition. *Philosophical Transactions of the Royal Society B* 366: 1050-1059.

Subbarayappa, B. V. 2001. The roots of ancient medicine: an historical outline. *Journal of Bioscience* (Indian Academy of Sciences) 26: 135-144.

Takahashi, K. and S. Yamanaka. 2006. Induction of pluripotent stem cells from mouse embryonic and adult fibroblast cultures by defined factors. *Cell* 126: 663-676.

Tamaki, M., Bang, J. W., Watanabe, T. et al. 2016. Night watch in one brain hemisphere during sleep associated with the first-night effect in humans. *Current Biology* 26: 1190-1194.

Tobaldini, E., Fiorelli, E. M., Solbiati, M. et al. 2018. Short sleep duration and cardiometabolic risk; from pathophysiology to clinical evidence. *Nature Reviews Cardiology*. doi:10.1038/s41569-018-0109-6.

Tomasello, M. 2018. How children come to understand false beliefs: a shared intentionality account. *PNAS* 115: 8491-8498.

Tountas, Y. 2009. The historical origins of the basic concepts of health promotion and education: the role of ancient Greek philosophy and medicine. *Health Promotion International* 24: 185-192.

Tripathi, M., Maheshwari, M. C., Jain, S. et al. 2000. Ayurvedic medicine and epilepsy. *Neurological Journal of South East Asia* 5: 1-4.

Tsujimoto, M., Komori, O. and S. Imura. 2016. Effect of lifespan and age on reproductive performance of the tardigrade Acutuncus antarcticus: minimal reproductive senescence. *Hydrobiologia* 772: 93-102.

Twenge, J. M., Krizan, Z. and G. Hisler. 2017. Decreases in self-reported sleep duration among U.S. adolescents 2009-2015 and association with new media screen time. *Sleep Medicine* 39: 47-53.

Van Leeuwen, E. J. C., Cronin, K. A. and D. B. M. Haun. 2018. Population-specific social dynamics in chimpanzees. *PNAS* 115: 11393-11400.

Van't Hof, A. E., Edmonds, N., Dalikova, M. et al. 2011. Industrial melanism in British peppered moths has a singular and recent mutational origin. *Science* 332:958-960.

Van't Hof, A. E., Campagne, P., Rigden, D. J. et al. 2016. The industrial melanism mutation in British peppered moths is a transposable element. *Nature* 534: 102-105.

Visscher, P. M., Wray, N. R., Zhang, Q. et al. 2017. 10 years of GWAS discovery: biology, function, and translation. *The American Journal of Human Genetics* 101: 5-22.

Wang, M-H., Marinotti, O., James, A. A. et al. 2010. Genome-wide patterns of gene expression during aging in the African malaria vector Anopheles gambiae. *PLOS ONE* 5(10). doi10.1371/journal.pone.0013359.

Weaver, I. C. G., D'Alessio, A. C., Brown, S. E. et al. 2007. The transcription factor nerve growth factor-inducible protein A mediates epigenetic programming: altering epigenetic marks by immediate–early genes. *Journal of Neuroscience* 27: 1756-1768.

Werner, M. S., Sieriebriennikov, B., loschko, T. et al. 2017. Environmental influence on Pristionchus pacificus mouth form through different culture methods. *Scientific Reports* 7:7207/doi: 10.1038/s41598-017-07455-7.

Westby, C. Theory of mind and language development and disorders. *Topics in Language Disorders* 34: 277-281.

West-Eberhard, M. J. 2019. Nutrition, the visceral immune system, and the evolutionary origins of pathogenic obesity. *PNAS* 116: 723-731.

Weyrich, L. S., Duchene, S., Soubrier, J. et al. 2017. Neanderthal behaviour, diet, and disease inferred from ancient DNA in dental calculus. *Nature* 544:357-361.

Wheaton, A. G., Liu, Y., Perry, G. S. et al. 2011. Effect of short sleep duration on daily activities-United States, 2005-2008. *Morbidity and Mortality Weekly Report* (United States) 60: 239-242.

Williams, S. A. and M. R. Shattuck. 2015. Ecology, longevity and naked mole rats: confounding effects of sociality? *Proceedings of the Royal Society* B 282: 20141664. doi. Org/10.1098/rspb.2014.1664.

Wong, K. 2018. Why did Homo sapiens alone survive to the modern era? *Scientific American* 319: 64-69.

Workneh, T., Emirie, G., Kaba, M. et al. 2018. Perceptions of health and illness among the Konso people of southwestern Ethiopia: Persistence and change. *Journal of Ethnobiology and Ethnomedicine* 14:18. doi.org/10.1186/s13002-018-0214-y.

Wray, N. R., Wijmenga, C., Sullivan, P. F. et al. 2018. Common disease is more complex than implied by the core gene omnigenic model. *Cell* 173: 1573-1580.

Yang, J., Huang, T., Petralia, F. et al. 2015. Synchronized age-related gene expression changes across multiple tissues in human and the link to complex diseases. *Scientific Reports* 5:15145/DOI:10.1038/srep15145.

Yetish, G., Kaplan, H., Gurven, M. et al. 2015. Natural sleep and its seasonal variations in three pre-industrial societies. *Current Biology* 25: 2862-2868.

Zhang, Y., Kim, M. S., Jia, B. et al. 2017. Hypothalamic stem cells control aging speed partly through exosomal miRNAs. *Nature* 548: 52-57.

ABOUT THE AUTHOR

Michael A. Singer
Emeritus Professor, Faculty of Health Sciences,
Queen's University,
Kingston, Ontario, Canada
Email: singerm@queensu.ca

Michael A. Singer graduated from University of Toronto Medical School in 1964. He did his Post Graduate training in Nephrology in Boston Massachusetts and Cambridge England. Joined Queen's University, Kingston, Ontario, Canada Faculty of Health Sciences in 1971. Retired from Queen's University in 1993 as Emeritus Professor.

INDEX

A

B

C

D

L

M

N

O

P

R

S

T

U

V

Related Nova Publications

Episodic Memory: Formation, Clinical Disorders and Role of Aging

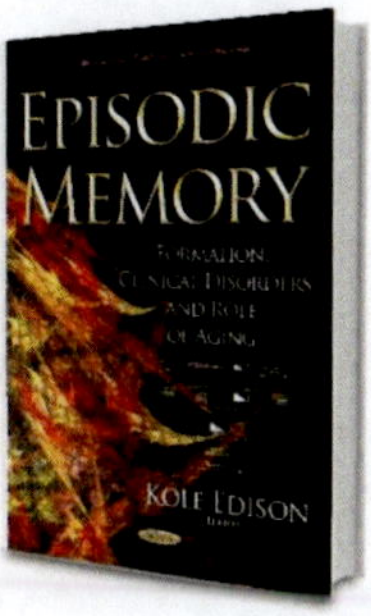

Editor: Kole Edison

Series: Neuroscience Research Progress

Book Description: This book focuses on episodic memory and the formation, clinical disorders and role of aging on episodic memory.

Hardcover ISBN: 978-1-63321-861-1
Retail Price: $192

Power and Aging: A Macro and Micro Analysis

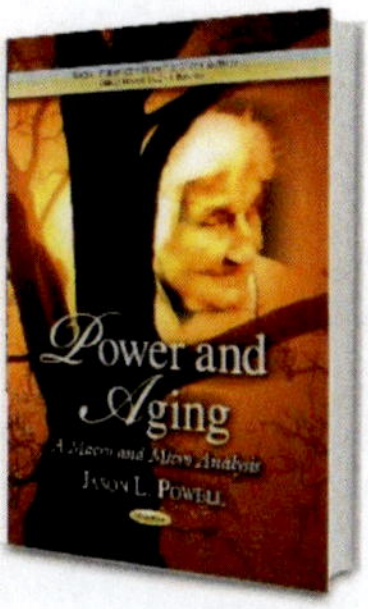

Author: Jason L. Powell

Series: Social Perspectives in the 21st Century

Book Description: This book examines the concept of power. It begins by pointing to its multi-dimensional definition and points to different sociological interpretations of its conception and social practice.

Softcover ISBN: 978-1-62948-534-8
Retail Price: $58

To see complete list of Nova publications, please visit our website at www.novapublishers.com

Related Nova Publications

Aging and Western Society: A Critical Approach

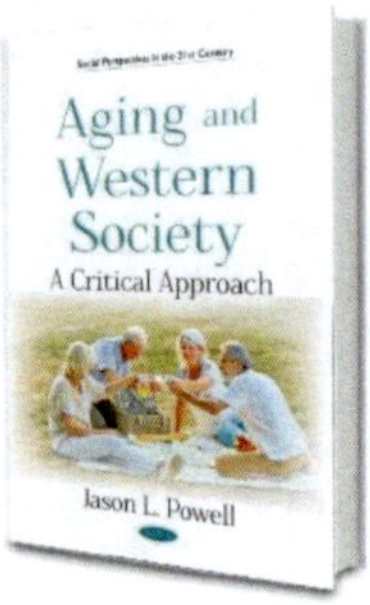

Author: Jason L. Powell

Series: Social Perspectives in the 21st Century

Book Description: This book is an unashamedly sociological excursion relating to the ageing process in Western society. It fundamentally questions assumptions and ideas around ageing, and where these ideas originate.

Softcover ISBN: 978-1-53613-844-3
Retail Price: $82

The Pilates Method: The Key to Successful Active Aging

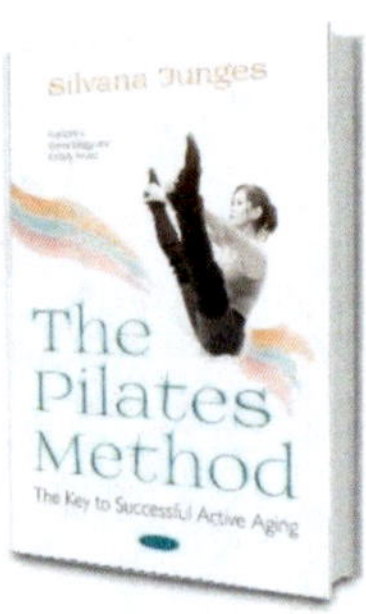

Author: Silvana Junges

Series: Geriatrics, Gerontology and Elderly Issues

Book Description: This book describes the origin of the Pilates method with its principles and foundations idealized by its creator, Joseph H Pilates. Based on his empirical studies and references of great Greek-Roman thinkers, Pilates was inspired to create a method for physical and mental health.

Softcover ISBN: 978-1-53612-174-2
Retail Price: $95

To see complete list of Nova publications, please visit our website at www.novapublishers.com